....
Lasers in Otorhinolaryngology, and in Head and Neck Surgery

Advances in Oto-Rhino-Laryngology

Vol. 49

Series Editor   *W. Arnold*, München

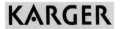

Basel · Freiburg · Paris · London · New York ·
New Delhi · Bangkok · Singapore · Tokyo · Sydney

4th International Symposium, Kiel, January 14–16, 1994

Lasers in Otorhinolaryngology, and in Head and Neck Surgery

Volume Editors

H. Rudert, Kiel
J.A. Werner, Kiel

56 figures, 1 in color, and 38 tables, 1995

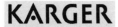

Basel · Freiburg · Paris · London · New York ·
New Delhi · Bangkok · Singapore · Tokyo · Sydney

....
Advances in Oto-Rhino-Laryngology

Library of Congress Cataloging-in-Publication Data
Lasers in otorhinolaryngology and in head and neck surgery: 4th international symposium, Kiel,
January 14–16, 1994 / volume editors, H. Rudert, J.A. Werner.
(Advances in oto-rhino-laryngology; vol. 49)
Includes bibliographical references and index.
1. Lasers in otolaryngology – Congresses.   2. Head – Laser surgery – Congresses.
3. Neck – Laser surgery – Congresses.   I. Rudert, H. (Heinrich), 1935–   .   II. Werner, J.A. (Jochen A.),
1958–   .   III. Series
[DNLM: 1. Otorhinolaryngologic Diseases – surgery – congresses.
2. Laser Surgery – congresses.   W1 AD701 v. 49 1995 / WV 168 L344 1995]
RF 51.5L374   1995   617.5'1059 – dc20

ISBN 3-8055-6087-7

Bibliographic Indices. This publication is listed in bibliographic services, including Current Contents® and Index Medicus.

Drug Dosage. The authors and the publisher have exerted every effort to ensure that drug selection and dosage set forth in this text are in accord with current recommendations and practice at the time of publication. However, in view of ongoing research, changes in government regulations, and the constant flow of information relating to drug therapy and drug reactions, the reader is urged to check the package insert for each drug for any change in indications and dosage and for added warnings and precautions. This is particularly important when the recommended agent is a new and/or infrequently employed drug.

© Copyright 1995 by S. Karger AG, P. O. Box, CH–4009 Basel (Switzerland)
Printed in Switzerland on acid-free paper by Thür AG Offsetdruck, Pratteln
ISBN 3–8055–6087–7

....

Contents

Laser Therapy in Plastic Surgery, and for Hemangiomas and Vascular Malformations

Otologic Applications of Laser Surgery

Nasal and Paranasal Applications of Laser Surgery

Laser Surgery for Benign Lesions in the Oral Cavity and Pharynx

Laser Surgery for Benign Laryngeal and Tracheal Lesions

Laser Surgery for Laryngeal Cancer

Preface

Medical laser techniques and technology develop very rapidly. Frequent updates are important to reflect the present state of the art. For this purpose, conferences on this subject have been held at the Department of Otorhinolaryngology, Head and Neck Surgery of the University of Kiel since 1985, and will be continued in the future.

The first two meetings in 1985 and 1988 dealt almost exclusively with applications of the CO_2 laser in otorhinolaryngology. During the third conference, in 1990, the use of the Nd:YAG laser was discussed, especially in the treatment of hemangiomas. This 4th Laser Congress presents an overview of six additional laser types already being used (for laser treatment of diseases of the middle and the inner ear, vascular malformations, diseases of the nasal cavity and the paranasal sinuses as well as benign and malignant tumors of the skin). Worldwide, transoral CO_2 laser surgery for laryngeal and hypopharyngeal cancer is a highly controversial topic. Long-term results show that it is justified to give transoral laser therapy an established place in the treatment of carcinomas, equal to conventional surgical partial resection of laryngeal or hypopharyngeal cancer. However, one has to avoid uncritical application of the CO_2 laser. It must satisfy the already complex criteria for conventional surgery of carcinomas.

Authors of the 4th Symposium of Lasers in Otorhinolaryngology, Head and Neck Surgery, Kiel, have been invited not only from Germany but also from Denmark, the Netherlands, Austria, Poland, Switzerland, Sweden, Hungary and the USA. They all have extensive experience with particular laser systems. The organizers of this meeting are proud to say that without exception everyone who was invited to participate did. Papers other than the invited lectures have been accepted to illustrate the situation of laser therapy outside the well-known centers.

The editors are delighted that almost all the speakers submitted their manuscripts for this book and for this we would like to thank them. The organizers would like to express their gratitude to the staff of Karger Publishers, Basel, for their spontaneous offer to publish all the lectures in the well-respected series *Advances in Oto-Rhino-Laryngology* in English, since there is presently no international up-to-date overview in which all the therapeutic applications of lasers in otorhinolaryngology, head and neck surgery are discussed.

Heinrich Rudert
Jochen A. Werner

Rudert H, Werner JA (eds): Lasers in Otorhinolaryngology, and in Head and Neck Surgery.
Adv Otorhinolaryngol. Basel, Karger, 1995, vol 49, pp 1–4

....

Tissue Effects of CO$_2$ Laser and Nd: YAG Laser

B.M. Lippert, J.A. Werner, H. Rudert

Department of Otolaryngology, Head and Neck Surgery at the
University of Kiel, Germany

Since the development of the first lasers by Maiman a whole variety of
different laser systems were established. In 1972, Strong and Jako [1] introduced the laser into otorhinolaryngology for endoscopic surgery of small vocal
cord carcinomas. Today, laser therapy is an established therapeutic concept in
the treatment of several benign and malignant diseases in ENT [2, 3].

Physical Tissue Effects

Tissue effects of laser beams depend on the specific qualities of the laser used and
the kind of tissue. Surgical use of laser beams requires a transformation of thermic energy
to coagulate and vaporize tissue. Thermic effects are mainly a result of absorption and distribution in the tissue [4].

Extension length in water of a CO$_2$ laser with a wavelength of 10.6 µm totals
0.03 mm. In this tissue level 90% of radiation energy will be absorbed [5]. In contrast to
CO$_2$ laser, absorption modalities of Nd:YAG lasers (wavelength: 1,064 µm) are mainly
due to tissue pigment content like hemoglobin [6]. Absorption of water-containing tissue
surfaces is small since radiation intrudes tissue deeper (up to 10 mm).

Primary Tissue Reaction

If laser beams hit tissue, tissue damage varies depending on the resulting temperature (>65 °C tissue coagulation; >150 °C tissue carbonization; >300 °C tissue vaporization). Lesions from vaporization are shaped like a crater. Often, damaged neighboring
zones to the tissue defect can be observed: the carbonization zone, the necrotic zone, and
the edematous zone [4, 7]. The amount of thermal-damaged zones varies depending on
the absorption criteria of the type of laser used, time of exposure, energy density of the laser, and tissue characteristics.

Cutting and Coagulation Qualities

The CO_2 laser is an excellent cutting device of highest precision and low thermic damage at the cutting edge. The cutting effect results from the thermic tissue reaction originating from the almost complete absorption of CO_2 laser beams by the water-containing tissue surface. The coagulation qualities of CO_2 lasers are low but while cutting a certain hemostatic effect can be observed up to a blood vessel diameter of 0.5 mm [2].

In contrast to CO_2 lasers, Nd:YAG laser beams penetrate tissues deeper during preparation and develop a uniform thermic coagulation. Good coagulation qualities allow occlusion of blood vessels up to a diameter of 5 mm [8]. High energy levels (>70 W) lead to a cutting effect by vaporization. Fine cuts as with the CO_2 laser cannot be achieved with this technique. In addition, cutting speed is low [9].

Influence on Blood and Lymphatic Vessels

Thermic effects of laser beams lead to several damaged zones of blood and lymphatic vessels. Only vessels reaching the carbonization zone will be sealed. This explains the lack of blood in CO_2 laser incisions. The Nd:YAG laser with its superior tissue penetration can occlude vessels of up to 5 mm in diameter by coagulation and shrinking. Damage to the capillaries is of crucial importance for wound healing. This laser-light-induced delay slows wound healing by 8–10 days. The determing factor is the extent of thermic damage along the cutting edges [10, 11].

The effect of laser beams on lymphatic vessels is of great interest in carcinoma surgery. Werner [12] could demonstrate that CO_2 and Nd:YAG lasers initially seal lymphatic vessels. In the carbonization zone lymphatic vessels cannot be detected, whereas some are still present in the edematous zone. Regeneration of lymphatic vessels starts about 8–10 days later than capillary proliferation, and is delayed after laser incision (10th postoperative day) if compared to a scalpel incision (4th postoperative day).

Influence of Several CO_2 Laser Parameters on Tissue Effects

The grade of thermic tissue damage is closely related to laser power, laser light radiated area and duration of exposure. Besides the laser power the influence of the beam diameter with regard to energy output density is of major interest. The focus diameter is mainly determined by the micromanipulator connected to the operation microscope rather than by the laser equipment itself [13]. The use of new micromanipulators allows a more than 60% reduced beam focus (>0.20 mm). A small laser beam can be used for incisions and preparation without a loss of laser energy density at the tissue level. In the continuous wave mode cutting qualities are higher using a reduced power output and laser light focus [14].

During the past years, the industry has developed new working modes for CO_2 lasers (in the literature often summarized as 'super-pulse wave mode') for better tissue protection with, at the same time, better cutting qualities. To put it simply, all CO_2 lasers use a sequence of single energy pulses of short pulse duration by high pulse frequency. Contrary to the continuous wave mode, the energy level is not constant. The tissue applicable energy density is many times higher than in the continuous wave mode [15]. The brief duration of the pulse is supposed to reduce the heating of the tissue and to allow better cooling in the pulse-free intervals. Histological examinations confirm the reduced thermic damage by using a high-energy CO_2 laser. In comparison to the continuous wave mode, carbonization and necrotic zones are significantly reduced [16].

For clinical purposes the use of CO_2 lasers demonstrate, under different parameters, several effects: The best quality of incision, hemostasis and differentiation of malignant and benign tissues in the continuous wave mode is achieved by using a reduced beam focus and energy output and makes reliable and precise tissue preparation possible. The high-energy working modes reduce carbonization and necrotic zones. An inhomogeneous and smaller necrotic zone increases intraoperative bleeding. In addition, tissue rupture makes the preparation of fine tissue structures more difficult [16, 17].

For clinical demand a laser as, for example, the excimer laser with total avoidance of necrotic zones is desirable. But ENT laser surgery on the mucosa cannot be the object of industrial research. The necrotic zone is the morphological substrate of modern, function-preserving carcinoma surgery. The necrotic zone is the reason that defects caused by laser surgery do not need to be covered.

References

1   Strong MS, Jako GJ: Laser-surgery in the larynx. Early clinical experience with continuous CO_2 laser. Ann Otol Rhinol Laryngol 1972;81:791–798.
2   Rudert H: Laser-Chirurgie in der HNO-Heilkunde. Laryngo Rhino Otol 1988;67:261–268.
3   Werner JA, Lippert BM, Godbersen GS, Rudert H: Die Hämangiombehandlung mit dem Neodym: Yttrium-Aluminium-Granat-Laser (Nd:YAG-Laser). Laryngo Rhino Otol 1992;71:388–395.
4   Helfmann J, Brodzinski T: Thermische Wirkungen; in Berlien HP, Müller G (eds): Angewandte Lasermedizin. Landsberg, Ecomed, 1989, pp II–3.3 1–8.
5   Bayly JG, Kartha VB, Stevens WH: The absorption spectra of liquid phase H_2O, DHO and D_2O from 0.7 μm. Infrared Phys 163;3:211–217.
6   Hardy JD, Hammel HT, Murgatroyd D: Spectral transmittance and reflectance of excised human skin. J Appl Physiol 1956;9:257–261.
7   Grossenbacher R: Laserchirurgie in der Oto-Rhino-Laryngologie; in Becker W, Boenninghaus H-G, Naumann H (eds): Aktuelle Oto-Rhino-Laryngologie, Heft 9. Stuttgart, Thieme, 1985, pp 16–22.

8   Keiditsch F, Hofstetter A, Zimmermann I, Stern J, Frank F, Babaryka: Histological investigation to substantiate the therapy of bladder tumors with the neodymium: YAG-laser. Laser Med Chir 1985;1:19–23.

9   Wallwiener D, Pollmann D, Stolz W, Kappler M, Bastert G, Krampe C: Die Nd:YAG-Kontakttechnik mit 'nackten' Glasfasern: lasertechnischer Background und Gewebeeffekte im Vergleich zur Präparation mit Saphirschneidespitzen. Laser Med Surg 1989;5:31–35.

10 Mecke H, Schünke M, Schnaidt S, Freys I, Semm K: Width of thermal damage after using the YAG contact laser for cutting biological tissue: Animal experimental investigation. Res Exp Med (Berl) 1991;1991:37–45.

11 Werner A, Lippert BM, Rudert H, Godbersen GS: Vergleichende Untersuchungen zur Revaskularisation der Schleimhaut des oberen Aerodigestivtraktes nach Skalpell-, CO_2- und Nd:YAG-Laserinzision. Eur Arch Oto Rhino Laryngol 1993;(suppl II):32–33.

12 Werner JA: Tierexperimentelle Untersuchungen zum Einfluss der CO_2- und Nd:YAG-Laserstrahlung auf die Lymphgefässe der Wangenschleimhaut. Laser Med 1992;2+3:141–142.

13 Werner JA, Lippert BM, Rudert H: Untersuchungen zu einem neuen Mikromanipulator in der CO_2-Lasermikrochirurgie; in Waidelich W, Waidelich R, Hofstetter A (eds): Laser in der Medizin (Laser in Medicine). Berlin, Springer, 1993, pp 343–344.

14 Lippert BM, Werner JA, Rudert H, Godbersen GS: Die Schnittqualität des CO_2-Lasers im Dauerstrich-, Superpuls-, Ultrapuls- und Pulserbetrieb: Eine experimentelle und klinische Untersuchung. Eur Arch Otorhinolaryngol 1993;(suppl II):31–32.

15 Badawy S, El Bakry MM, Baggish MS: Comparative study of continuous and pulsed CO_2 laser on tissue healing and fertility outcome in tubal anastomosis. Fertil Steril 1987;47:843–847.

16 Lippert BM, Werner JA, Rudert H: Experimentelle und klinische Untersuchungen zur Schnittqualität des CO_2-Lasers bei unterschiedlichen Betriebsformen; in Waidelich W, Waidelich R, Hofstetter A (eds): Laser in der Medizin (Laser in Medicine). Berlin, Springer, 1993, pp 341–342.

17 Werner JA, Rudert H: CO_2- und Nd:YAG-Laser: Beschreibung und Vergleich ihres Wirkungsgrades am biologischen Gewebe. Eur Arch Otorhinolaryngol 1989;(suppl II):214–215.

Dr. B.M. Lippert, Department of Otorhinolaryngology, Head and Neck Surgery,
University of Kiel, Arnold-Heller-Strasse 14, D–24105 Kiel (Germany)

Rudert H, Werner JA (eds): Lasers in Otorhinolaryngology, and in Head and Neck Surgery.
Adv Otorhinolaryngol. Basel, Karger, 1995, vol 49, pp 5–7

....

In vivo Models for Studies of Laser Effects on Blood Vessels

K. Schwager [a], *M. Waner* [b], *S. Flock* [b]

[a] Universitätsklinik und Poliklinik für Hals-, Nasen- und Ohrenkranke Würzburg
   (Direktor: Prof. *J. Helms*), Germany;
[b] Department of Otolaryngology, Head and Neck Surgery (Head: Prof. *J.Y. Suen*),
   University of Arkansas, Little Rock, Ark., USA

Since laser procedures have become more and more established in medicine, in vivo models are necessary to study the laser-tissue interaction. A special interest is in the reaction of vascular tissue, especially in the treatment of vascular lesions. Lasers that emit light of a wavelength that is absorbed by oxyhemoglobin and less by the melanin of the skin are in use to treat vascular lesions such as hemangiomas and port wine stains. The wavelength used initially was the green-blue of the Argon laser, but more recently yellow light at the wavelength of 575–585 nm was introduced to treat these lesions [1, 2]. Two major questions arise concerning laser tissue interaction. First, what happens to the overlying skin, and, second, what happens to the vessel itself. Four models will be presented, using tissue from different regions of the albino rat.

In vivo Models

The Rat Ear
The rat ear is a useful model to study vascular reactions and the reaction of the overlying skin as well. Here can be seen major feeding vessels branching into smaller vessels which terminate as an arcade at the margin of the ear. After laser treatment, the damage to the tissue and the following healing can be observed.

Rat Dorsal Skin-Flap Window-Chamber Model
This model was first utilized for studies in photodynamic therapy [3, 4]. The dorsum is shaved and the dorsal skin fold is fixed by a metal framework. The skin on one side is removed and the subcutaneous tissue which is covered with glass allows a direct study of

subcutaneous tissue reactions. Because the animals tolerate this device very well, long-term and healing studies can also be performed [5, 6].

Rat Colon (Cecum) Model

A greater number and more varied size of vessels for experimentation can be found in the colon such as the cecum of the rat [7]. The shaved abdomen of the anesthetized animal is opened by means of a midline incision and the cecum carefully luxated with cotton tips. The cecum is positioned on the animal and surrounded by gauze and covered with a glass microscope slide which serves to minimize movement of the cecum. The gauze and the specimen are kept moist using body temperature 0.9% saline solution. Irradiation of the vessels takes place through the glass slide.

The size of the vessels is very different. From central vessels of the diameter of several hundred micrometers to capillaries there is a wide variety in vessel size. In the same field, there are always many vessels of the same size, and every vein is accompanied by an artery.

Isolated Vessels (Femoral Artery)

Sometimes it is necessary to study the irradiation on single, even bigger vessels. The femoral artery is a possible vessel model for this [8]. The animal is first brought into the supine position and a cut is made in the groin. The bundle of the femoral nerve, artery and vein is dissected and separated under the microscope. Care is taken to remove all the adjacent connective tissue of the vessel. The separated vessel is then isolated from the surrounding tissue by means of a plastic background sheet. The chamber created by the skin edges of the cut is filled with body temperature 0.9% saline solution.

Discussion

Two of the presented models are useful for follow-up and healing studies: the ear model [9], and the rat dorsal skin-flap window-chamber model. After irradiation, which is always performed in the anesthetized animal, the animals can be followed up for the upcoming repair process. Even the animals for the dorsal frame work will tolerate this [4].

The cecum model and the studies on single vessels like the femoral artery can only be used to do studies on the anesthetized animal and after the experiment the animal has to be sacrificed. The ear model offers the opportunity to study the dermal reaction as well [9]. In yellow light application, modeling the treatment of vascular lesions, it is necessary to study both the effects on the vascular tissue and the side effects to the overlying skin.

A wide variety of different vessel sizes can be experimented with in the cecum model. Certain phenomena can be observed on several vessels of the same size, and can be repeated easily. To show a certain effect on a single vessel, it is sometimes necessary to use a bigger vessel, that can easily be dissected from its surrounding tissue; in studies with a nanosecond pulsed light from a frequency doubled Nd:YAG laser, the rupture of the side opposite to the irradiation was noticed. Using the femoral artery as a single-vessel model, this phenomenon which is probably caused by shockwaves could be demonstrated and confirmed [8].

Conclusion

When looking for an in vivo model for vascular laser tissue reaction, one has to know that all these models have certain disadvantages. Before starting an experimental setup, it should be recognized that while a particular model may be suitable to answer a specific question, it may not adequately address other issues. For that reason, it is often necessary to use different models to assess different aspects of laser tissue interaction.

References

1   Anderson RR, Jaenicke KF, Parrish JA: Mechanisms of selective vascular changes caused by dye lasers. Lasers Surg Med 1983;3:211–215.
2   Anderson RR, Parrish JA: Selective photothermiolysis: Precise microsurgery by selective absorption of pulsed radiation. Science 1983;220:524–527.
3   Papenfuss HD, Gross JF, Intaglietta M, Treese FA: A transparent access chamber for the rat dorsal skin fold. Microvasc Res 1979;18:311–318.
4   Stern SJ, Flock S, Small S, Thomsen S, Jaques S: An implantable tumor-window chamber model for the study of photodynamic therapy. Otolaryngol Head Neck Surg 1991;105:556–566.
5   Flock S, Waner M, McGrew B, Colvin GB, Montague D: A comparison of the treatment of vascular lesions with the copper vapor laser and flashlamp-pumped dye laser, in Anderson RR, Bass LS, Shapshay SM, Whirte JV, White RA (eds): Lasers in Otolaryngology, Dermatology, and Tissue Welding. Proc SPIE 1992;1646;98–106.
6   Flock S, Waner M, Schwager K, McGrew B, Montague D: The response of blood vessels to radiation by four different vascular lesion lasers: Argon dye, copper-vapor, flashlamp-dye and frequency-doubled Nd:YAG-dye. Proc Int Conf Photodynamic Therapy and Medical Laser Applications, vol ICS 1011, Milan 1992. Amsterdam, Elsevier, 1992.
7   Schwager K, Flock S, Waner M: Das Coecum der Ratte als vaskuläres Modell bei der Anwendung von nanosekundengepulstem Laserlicht. Eur Arch ORL 1993;(suppl 1993/II):33.
8   Schwager K, Flock S, Waner M: Effects of nanosecond pulsed laser light (577 nm) from a Q-switched frequency-doubled Nd:YAG-dye laser on experimental vascular tissue; in Anderson RR, Bass LS, Shapshay SM, Whirte JV, White RA (eds): Lasers in Otolaryngology, Dermatology, and Tissue Welding, Proc SPIE 1993;1876:113–119.
9   Landthaler M, Haina D, Brunner R, Waidelich W, Braun-Falco: Effects of argon, dye and Nd: Yag lasers on epidermis, dermis and venous vessels. Lasers Surg Med 1986;6:87–93.

Dr. K. Schwager, Universitätsklinik und Poliklinik für Hals-, Nasen- und Ohrenkranke Würzburg, D–97080 Würzburg (Germany)

Rudert H, Werner JA (eds): Lasers in Otorhinolaryngology, and in Head and Neck Surgery.
Adv Otorhinolaryngol. Basel, Karger, 1995, vol 49, pp 8–14

....

Characteristic Features of Wound Healing in Laser-Induced Incisions

M. Schünke[a], *C. Krüss*[b], *H. Mecke*[c], *J.A. Werner*[d]

[a] Anatomisches Institut der Universität Kiel;
[b] Westerland/Sylt;
[c] Auguste-Viktoria-Krankenhaus Berlin;
[d] Klinik für Hals-, Nasen-, Ohrenheilkunde, Kopf- und Halschirurgie der Universität
Kiel, Deutschland

Laser surgery has become a widely used clinical treatment especially in otorhinolaryngology [1]. From the medically useful lasers the neodymium YAG and the carbon dioxide (CO_2) lasers are the most widely used. Whereas the Nd:YAG laser has good coagulation properties, the CO_2 laser is predominantly employed for cutting. As the effect of CO_2 laser on tissue is purely thermal, precise excisions have been claimed as one of the major advantages of CO_2 laser. There is better visualization with lack of bleeding and, in addition, clinical experience has shown that laser-treated tissue heals with less postoperative pain. However, secondary tissue reactions and delayed healing limit its use.

General Features of Cellular Events in Normal Wound Healing

The result of an injury, the fresh wound, sets off a number of processes in the organism which are all directed towards the final purpose of repair [2]. Regardless of the type of wound, three characteristic phases of wound healing can be differentiated: (a) The inflammatory or exudative phase, (b) the proliferate or regenerative phase, and (c) the repair phase. These phases differ in terms of how long they last, but they also partially overlap (fig. 1).

During the *exudative phase* blood and lymph escape into the wound cavity initiating the activation of the clotting system. The further course of wound healing is primarily activated by the signals that are given off during this phase.

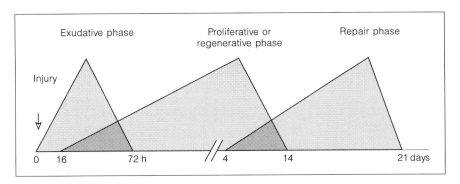

Fig. 1. Time course of normal wound healing. From Wokalek [2].

Migration of inflammatory cells (polymorphonuclear neutrophilic granulocytes, monocytes, macrophages, lymphocytes and mast cells) into the coagulum, phagocytosis of necrotic debris and release of chemotactic substances (PDGF, TFG-β) are the major events. The beginning of this phase is marked by catabolism.

The *proliferate* or *regenerative phase* is above all characterized by increased fibroblast activity and the acceleration of cell division as well as the proliferation of blood vessels. During this anabolic peroid granulation tissue is formed.

The *repair phase* is characterized by the formation of new connective tissue, the activity of myofibroblasts (wound contraction), the maturing of collagen and the reepithelialization of the wound.

Possible Mechanism of Laser-Induced Delay in Wound Healing

In agreement with several experimental investigations [3–5], we found the following reasons to be responsible for delayed wound healing observed after laser incisions. For comparison, scalpel incisions in rat mouth mucosa (fig. 2, 3) were also studied.

Carbonization. The mechanism of tissue incision with the CO_2 laser is vaporization of tissue water and rapid expansion causing cell disruption. Immediate postoperative observation revealed a crater-shaped wound with its walls and floor covered with carbonized tissue. However, charred debris acts as a foreign body in the laser wound and lead to granuloma with increased scar formation (fig. 3).

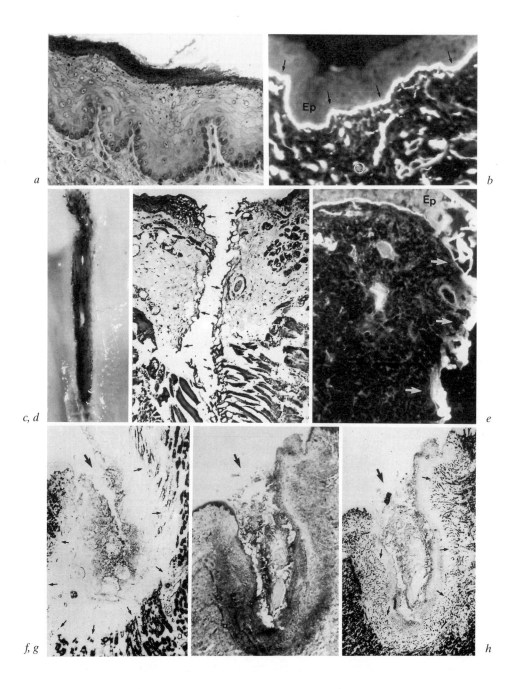

a

b

c, d

e

f, g

h

Ep

Ep

Schünke/Krüss/Mecke/Werner

Thermal Necrosis. During laser treatment the laser wound margin undergoes thermal necrosis. However, in the immediate laser wound necrotic tissue is limited to a very narrow zone, usually ranging from 300 to 600 μm (fig. 2). There is evidence of endothelial damage and thrombosis of the capillaries and smaller vessels as revealed from the complete negative immunohistochemical staining for laminin throughout the entire necrotic tissue. As laminin is one of the major components of basement membranes, we suppose that thermal influence could alter basement membrane composition with subsequent reduction of permeability.

Inflammatory Cell Infiltration and Capillary Proliferation. Due to laser-induced bloodless surgery there is no blood clot sealing the laser wound within a few hours after surgery. Therefore, platelets do not aggregate in the wound and release of biologically active factors, including the platelet-derived growth factor (PDGF), does not take place. For example, PDGF stimulates cell replication and is one of the most potent chemoattractants known [6]. Due to the delayed inflammatory cell infiltration, removal of necrotic material is also slowed down. Therefore, beginning of neovascularization proceeds much slower as compared to bleeding wounds [10].

Granulation Tissue Formation. The formation of granulation tissue depends mainly on the activity of fibroblasts producing extracellular matrix components (type III collagen, glycosaminoglycans). Due to a delayed immigration of fibroblasts and a decreased cell activity, formation of granulation tissue occurs more slowly as compared to scalpel incisions (fig. 2).

Contraction of Wound Edges. Myofibroblasts obviously do not play a major role in laser wound closure as the wounds heal without any observable contraction [7]. Histological sections on postoperative day 15 (fig. 3) revealed only few myofibroblasts resulting in decreased wound contraction and thus also delayed wound healing considerably.

Fig. 2. a Histological section of normal mouth mucosa stained with toluidinblue. *b* Frozen section of normal mouth mucosa immunostained with an antilaminin antibody, note the bright staining of basement membranes (arrows) beneath the epidermis (Ep) and around the capillaries. *c* Macroscopic view of a CO_2 laser wound shortly after laser incision (power density of approximately 4,000 W/cm^2 per unit beam area). *d* Corresponding histological section of (*c*), note the carbonised wound edges (arrows). *e* Immunofluorescence staining for laminin in the laser wound 1 day after surgery, nonspecific fluorescence of carbonized material. Ep = Epidermis. *f* ATPase-negative necrotic zone (arrows). *g* Inflammatory cell infiltration with acid phosphatase-positive cells within the laser wound 5 days after surgery. *h* Capillary proliferation (arrows) as seen by positive endothelial ATPase-reaction in a 5-day-old laser wound. $a \times 120$. $b \times 60$. $c \times 5$. $d \times 35$. $e \times 60$. $f \times 30$. $g \times 30$. $h \times 30$.

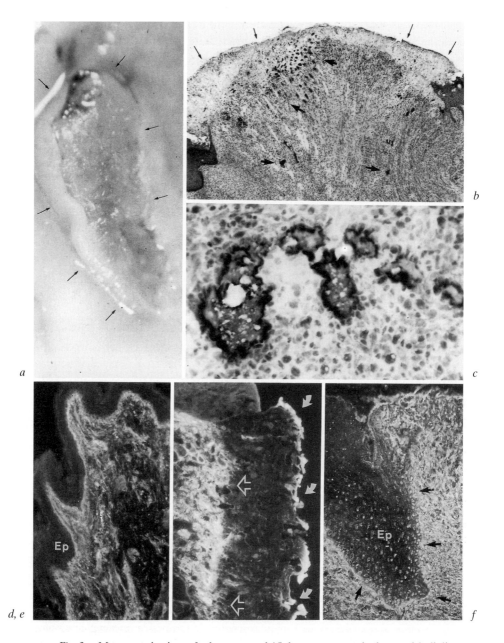

Fig. 3. a Macroscopic view of a laser wound 15 days postoperatively, reepithelialization has not yet taken place (arrows point at the wound edge). *b* Corresponding histological section of (*a*) shows nonepithelialized wound surface (arrows) and granulation tissue
with charred debris (big arrows). *c* Charred debris act as foreign bodies and lead to granuloma. *d* Control section with normal fibronectin distribution, especially beneath the epi-

Fibronectin Deficiency. Fibronectin occurs in high amounts in plasma (300 µg/ml) and is introduced into the wound with influx of blood. It also appears to be one of the principal chemoattractants secreted by macrophages. Fibronectin (MG = 440,000 daltons) is a fibrillar glycoprotein and interacts with cells important to wound healing including platelets, neutrophilic granulocytes, monocytes, endothelial cells, and epidermal cells [8]. In addition, it binds to fibrin and various matrix components and therefore it is unlikely that the intact molecule is able to penetrate into the adjacent tissue [9, 10]. We suppose that the initial lack of fibronectin is one of the major reasons for a delayed wound healing.

Reepithelialization. Another important role of fibronectin during cutaneous repair is to provide the substratum for keratinocyte migration [11]. It is presumed that plasma fibronectin is positivily involved in the adhesion and extension of epithelial cells in the process of reepithelialization. Keratinocytes become adhesive toward fibronectin under wound healing conditions [12] and begin to express specific fibronectin receptors (α_3/β_1-integrins). However, it is also possible that activation of keratinocytes leads to a relocalization of the cell-cell adhesion receptors mediating events involving cell-matrix interactions [13, 14]. On the fibronectin matrix, keratinocyte migration increases and, for example, topical application of fibronectin has been shown to promote epithelialization of nonhealing venous stasis ulcers [15, 16].

Conclusions

From our studies it can be concluded that wound healing appears to be delayed in laser incisions as compared to scalpel incisions. This is mainly due to carbonization of the wound margins, thermal necrosis, delayed removal of necrotic material, diminished fibroblast activity and formation of granulation tissue and a retarded initiation of reepithelialization. One of the main reasons, however, is the bloodless wound with absence of plasma fibronectin depositions.

dermis (Ep). *e* Immediately after surgery, fibronectin immunostaining of the necrotic zone is negative, intensive fibronectin deposition in the underlying connective tissue (empty arrows), nonspecific fluorescence of carbonized tissue (arrows). *f* Reepithelialization phase, immunopositive, basal keratinocytes in the newly formed epidermis (Ep) next to the basement membrane (arrows). *d–f* Frozen sections stained with FITC-conjugated antimouse fibronectin antibodies: $a \times 10$. $b \times 35$. $c \times 200$. $d \times 30$. $e \times 50$. $f \times 90$.

References

1   Rudert H: Laser-Chirurgie in der HNO-Heilkunde. Laryngo Rhino Otol 1988;67:261–268.
2   Wokalek H: Cellular events in wound healing. Crit Rev Biocomp 1988;4:209–246.
3   Luomanen M, Meurman JH, Lehto VP: Extracellular matrix in healing CO_2 laser incision wound. J Oral Pathol 1987;16:322–331.
4   Basu MK, Frame JW, Rhys Evans PH: Wound healing follow partial glossectomy using CO_2 laser, diathermy and scalpel: A histological study in rats. J Laryngol Otol 1988;102:322–327.
5   Watanabe IS, Lopes RA, Liberti EA, Azeredo RA, Takakura CH, Goldenberg S: Light and scanning electron microscopic studies of the effects of CO_2 laser on the palatine mucosa of rats. Z Mikros Anat Forsch 1989;103:925–935.
6   Ross R, Glomset J, Kariya B, Harker L: A platelet-dependent serum factor that stimulates the proliferation of arterial smooth muscle cells in vitro. Proc Natl Acad Sci USA 1974;71:1207–1210.
7   Finesmith TH, Broadly KN, Davidson JM: Fibroblasts from wounds of different stages of repair vary in their ability to contract a collagen gel in response to growth factors. J Cell Physiol 1990;144:99–107.
8   Wysocki AB: Fibronectin in acute and chronic wounds. J Et Nurs 1992;19:166–170.
9   Casscells W, Kimura H, Sanchez JA, Yu ZX, Ferans VJ: Immunhistochemical study of fibronectin in experimental myocardial infarction. Am J Pathol 1990;137:801–810.
10 Grinnell F: Fibronectin and wound healing. J Cell Biochem 1984;26:107–116.
11 Pospisilova J, Riebelova V: Fibronectin: Its significance in wound epithelialization. Acta Chir Plast 1986;28:96–102.
12 Clark RAF: Fibronectin matrix deposition and fibronectin receptor expression in healing and normal skin. J Invest Dermatol 1990;94:128–134.
13 Larjava H: Expression of beta-1 integrins in normal human keratinocytes. Am J Med Sci 1991;301:63–68.
14 Adams JC, Watt FM: Changes in keratinocyte adhesion during terminal differentiation: Reduction in fibronectin binding precede α_5/β_1-integrin in loss from the cell surface. Cell 1990;63: 425–435.
15 Nagelschmidt M, Fischer H, Engelhardt GH: Reversal of gelatin-impaired-wound healing in rats by exogenous fibronectin. J Surg Res 1992;53:490–494.
16 Kim KS, Oh JS, Kim IS, Jo JS: Clinical efficacy of topical homologous fibronectin in persistent corneal epithelial disorders. Korean J Ophthalmol 1992;6:12–18.

Prof. Dr. Dr. Michael Schünke, Anatomisches Institut der Christian-Albrechts-Universität zu Kiel, Olshausenstraße 40, D–24098 Kiel (Germany)

Rudert H, Werner JA (eds): Lasers in Otorhinolaryngology, and in Head and Neck Surgery.
Adv Otorhinolaryngol. Basel, Karger, 1995, vol 49, pp 15–19

....

Anesthesiological Problems of Endolaryngeal and Endotracheal Laser Surgery

W. Jeckström[a], *J. Wawersik*[a], *P. Hoffmann*[b], *J.A. Werner*[b],
B.M. Lippert[b], *B. Christiansen*[c], *R. Paustian*[d], *U. Sowada*[d]

[a] Klinik für Anästhesiologie und Operative Intensivmedizin;
[b] Klinik für Hals-, Nasen-, Ohrenheilkunde, Kopf- und Halschirurgie;
[c] Institut für Hygiene und Umweltmedizin im Klinikum der Christian-Albrechts-
   Universität Kiel;
[d] Institut für Feinwerktechnik, Fachbereich Technik, Fachhochschule Kiel,
   Deutschland

Laser surgery of the upper aerodigestive tract can cause a collision of the interests of the surgeon and the anesthesiologist. The main problems are the potential effect of the laser on the tube and the narrow anatomic situation. A modification of regular anesthesiological techniques is therefore necessary with respect to the physical properties of the tube, the ventilation technique, the anesthetic gases and the relaxation.

Material and Methods

In the past 5 years more than 1,200 laser surgical operations in the upper aerodigestive tract were performed in total intravenous anesthesia. The age of patients ranged from 3 months to 88 years.

The following special laser tubes were tested experimentally: Norton, Mallinckrodt Laser-Flex™, Hennef, Medimex Fome Cuf, Hamburg; Xomed-Treace Laser-Shield II™, Jacksonville. The experiments were performed with a CO_2 laser Sharplan 1055S, Freising, in a continuous-wave mode through an operating microscope with a 400-mm objective lense.

(1) To evaluate the noninflammability of laser tubes, the CO_2 laser beam was directed to the surface of the tubes at a right angle with a laser power of 30 W (focal diameter 0.25 mm) for 2 min.

(2) Airway resistance was measured at a constant flow of 230 ml/s in tubes with an inner diameter (ID) of 6 mm. These values correspond to the situation in a healthy adult. For comparison, a conventional PVC tube, Intermediate Trachealtube Mallinckrodt (Hennef; ID 6 mm) was examined.

(3) To study the reflection of the tubes the following experiment was performed: CO_2 laser light with a laser power of 6 W (focal diameter 0.25 mm) was applied on the surface of laser tubes (ID 6 mm) with an angle of 45°. The reflected radiation was measured with a thermocolumn containing a large number of separate thermo-elements.

(4) Tubeless ventilation was performed in cases where the intubation tube hindered the surgeon. During proximal jet ventilation the tip of the jet needle is placed in front of the larynx but inside the laryngoscope [1]. An alternative method is the distal jet ventilation technique where the tip of the jet needle is placed below the glottic area in the subglottis. Intrathoracic pressures can get dangerously high with this technique. For early detection of high intratracheal pressure, this was monitored through a second channel of the jet needle.

(5) Laser plume was evaluated regarding its content of bacteria. Swabs were taken from the surface of tumor in 5 patients who underwent laser surgery for carcinoma of the larynx. A filter (PALL Ultipor BB50, London) was installed right behind the metal suction which was inserted into the laryngoscope. This filter was connected to the suction pump (Vaculas AS10, Limmer Medical Technology, Appen) with a flow of 200 liters/min. Different filters were used for suction with and without laser surgery for 15 min each. Both of the sides that faced the patient and the sides that faced the suction pump were cultured in the microbiological laboratory.

Results

(1) All laser tubes were not inflammable in the protected part.

(2) The airway resistance of the tubes was as follows: Mallinckrodt 65.2 $mbar \times /l^{-1} \times sec^{-1}$, Medimax 47.8 $mbar \times /l^{-1} \times sec^{-1}$, Norton, Xomed and PVC 34.7 $mbar \times /l^{-1} \times sec^{-1}$.

(3) The highest reflected radiation values were measured in the Norton tube with 1.96 mW, followed by the Mallinckrodt laser tube (1.64 mW). They were much lower in the Medimex tube (0.14 mW) and the Xomed tube (0.08 mW).

(4) Jet ventilation was performed in 127 patients. In 5 of these patients sufficient ventilation was not possible because the jet cannula could not be placed properly through the microlaryngoscope due to the individual anatomy. No other complications were observed.

(5) During laser surgery bacteriological studies could show contamination in all filter sides that faced the patients. No contamination was found on the filter sides which faced the suction pump. In 4 of 5 patients the same bacteria as in the swabs were found. No bacteria were detected in the filters where the suction was active without the laser.

Discussion

The worst anesthesiological complication of laser surgery of the upper aerodigestive tract is tube fire induced by the laser. It is observed with an incidence varying between 0.4 and 1.5% [2]. No tube fires occurred in more than 1,200 laser surgical operations in the upper aerodigestive tract performed at the Department of Otorhinolaryngology at the University of Kiel. Today, special laser tubes are available which are noninflammable in the protected part. This, however, is not true for the cuff area and the tip of the laser tube. Burning of the cuff on the other hand seems very unlikely since the cuff is filled with saline solution and can be protected by moistened gauze pads.

One problem of laser tubes is the airway resistance. We surprisingly found that higher ventilation pressures are necessary in the Mallinckrodt and Medimex laser tube. This is especially problematic since many of our patients also suffer from chronic respiratory diseases with an increased airway resistance which adds to the increased airway resistance of the laser tube. High intrathoracic pressures may result which can cause complications with ventilation and circulation.

Another problem may result from the physical effect of the laser on the surface of the laser tube. The laser tube can reflect or absorb the laser radiation very differently. The reflection of laser radiation can cause unintended and accidental burns of the tissue. The lowest reflection was found for the Xomed tube.

Regular PVC or rubber tubes are still used in many cases to save the expense of costly laser tubes. These tubes can be ignited by a focused laser beam during ventilation with 100% oxygen or a mixture of nitrous oxide and oxygen. Therefore, the use of oxygen-air or oxygen-helium mixtures with a total inspired oxygen concentration of less than 40% has been advocated [3]. The availability of intravenous anesthesia makes the use of anesthetic gases like halothane, isoflurane and enflurane unnecessary. They can cause further problems because they may contaminate the operating room during tubeless ventilation and because they can be decomposed at very high temperatures into substances of unknown pharmacological effects. Ventilation through an intubation tube should generally be the method of choice. However, it cannot be used if it interferes with adequate surgical exposure, e.g. in children or in surgery of the dorsal larynx. In these cases tubeless ventilation techniques are required. Methods used today are the proximal and distal jet ventilation. These methods have been used successfully and without complications at our department. Another possibility is the use of the Hayek cuirass oscillator [4]. All tubeless ventilation techniques have specific disadvantages. Most important is the fact that the patient is not protected against aspiration.

Another problem is the laser plume generated by the laser beam when vaporizing the tissue at temperatures higher than 400 °C. The plume contains particles with a diameter ranging from 0.1 to more than 9 µm which can transfer microorganisms [5]. Fourteen percent of the laser surgically excised tissue mass can be found in the laser plume as particulate debris [6]. Jet ventilation, especially proximal jet ventilation, can blow the smoke into the lung of the patient but also into the operating room. If inhaled, the majority of these smoke particles would be deposited in the lung at the level of the alveoli. Therefore, a sufficient plume evacuation system (flow >200 liters/min) with adequate filters (pore size <0.1 µm) must be available. Another way to avoid contamination is the interruption of ventilation during activation of the laser. Operation in apnea is especially useful when operating on the trachea and the bronchial system.

Complete relaxation is essential during laser surgical procedures to avoid accidental damage of healthy and functional tissue. Atracurium and norcuronium do not always sufficiently suppress muscle movements. Succinylcholine is at present the substance of choice in laryngeal operations because it causes complete relaxation. It does, however, have many adverse effects such as myoglobinemia, hyperkaliemia, arrhythmia and postoperative muscle pain. The most important problem is the hangover relaxation which cannot be antagonized so that some patients require prolonged controlled ventilation.

Laser surgery of the upper aerodigestive tract requires an intensified monitoring. Online video monitoring is essential so that the anesthesiologist can immediately detect any hazards interfering with the ventilation. The necessity to ventilate with the lowest possible FIO_2 affords transcutaneous oxygen saturation measurement. To complete the technical surveillance the following parameters should also be measured: FIO_2, ECG, blood pressure, relaxation, breathing pressure and exspired CO_2 concentration.

Conclusion

Laser surgery in the upper aerodigestive tract necessitates a modification of anesthesiological techniques. Most important is the use of a laser tube which is the only protection against tube fires. This is especially true if the intubation tube is placed very close to the actual laser incision or if the surgeon lacks profound experience with the laser. Anesthetic gases (no nitrous oxide but air-oxygen or helium-oxygen with $FIO_2 < 40\%$) and intraoperative monitoring (transcutaneous oxygen saturation, online video) have to be adapted to the situation during laser surgery. For short operations laser excision in apnea is sufficient. Tubeless ventilation techniques like jet ventilation or Hayek cuirass oscillator should be restricted to special cases.

Compliance with the recommended modifications makes laser surgery a safe method. The basis for successful laser surgery in the upper aerodigestive tract, however, is the trustful team approach between the anesthesiologist and the surgeon.

References

1 Jeckström W, Wawersik J, Werner JA: Narkosetechnik bei laserchirurgischen Eingriffen im Kehlkopfbereich. HNO 1992;40:28–32.
2 Heine P, Axhausen M: Anästhesie und Laserchirurgie im Hals-Nasen-Ohrenbereich. Anaesthesist 1988;37:10–18.
3 Sosis MB, Braverman B: Prevention of cautery-induced airway fires with special endotracheal tubes. Anesth Analg 1993;77:846–847.
4 Dilkes MG, McNeill JM, Hill AC, Monks PS, McKelvie P, Hollamby RG: The Hayek oscillator: A new method of ventilation in microlaryngeal surgery. Ann Otol Rhinol Laryngol 1993;102; 455–458.
5 Ernst FH: Potential hazards of vaporized byproducts: A need for precautions. J Oral Maxillofac Surg 1992;50:313.
6 Mahashi S, Jako GJ, Inze J, Strong MS, Vaughn CW: Laser surgery on otolaryngology, interaction of CO_2 laser and soft tissue. Ann NY Acad Sci 1975;267:263–294.

Dr. Werner Jeckström, Klinik für Anästhesiologie und Operative Intensivmedizin, Schwanenweg 21, D–24105 Kiel (Germany)

Rudert H, Werner JA (eds): Lasers in Otorhinolaryngology, and in Head and Neck Surgery.
Adv Otorhinolaryngol. Basel, Karger, 1995, vol 49, pp 20–22

....

Problems Caused by Laser Plume, Especially Considering Laser Microlaryngoscopy

Wolfgang Wöllmer

Universitäts-HNO-Klinik (Direktor: Prof. *U. Koch*), Universitätskrankenhaus
Eppendorf, Hamburg, Deutschland

Pyrolysis products emanating from the site of impact of the laser beam
during laser surgery, commonly called laser plume, obstruct the view of the operation field and bother the staff by their unpleasant smell. Moreover, some
publications [1–6] indicate that the plume may contain toxic chemical substances or even infectious particles. Starting in 1992, this problem is being investigated systematically in a EUREKA joint project [8] by four German institutions, sponsored by the German Minister of Research and Technology:
(1) Freie Universität Berlin, University Hospital Steglitz, Institute of Medi-
    cal/Technical Physics and Laser Medicine in cooperation with the Laser-
    Medizin-Zentrum GmbH, Berlin.
(2) Humboldt-Universität Berlin, University Hospital Charité and Universi-
    tät der Bundeswehr Munich, Institute of Physics.
(3) Universität Hamburg, University Hospital Eppendorf, Ear Nose and
    Throat Clinic.
(4) Universität Ulm, Institute of Industrial and Social Medicine, and Institute
    of Laser Technologies in Medicine.
  Among the examined fields of medical laser application laser microlaryngoscopy demands special consideration, since the plume arises within the aerodigestive tract of the patient and hence implies an increased risk of exposition
to possibly infectious virus compounds or other aerosol particles as well as
short-lived, chemically aggressive reaction products [14].
  Laser plume can largely be removed by appropriate evacuators. Test of
different models and definition of essential properties of such apparatus are
also subjects of the joint project [7]. It turns out that the design of the suction
nozzle plays an important role for the efficiency of the plume removal [17].

New developments of microlaryngoscopic devices under this aspect have recently been presented [20]. Effective filtering of the plume within the evacuation system is of major importance [18]. After use, a fraction of the plume is found condensed in the suction tubes which under the microscope appears as droplets and particles. Their consistency is one of the priority subjects of the joint project being investigated with different methods of aerosol research [15]. The main topic certainly is the gas chromatographic-mass spectrometric analysis of small molecules and volatile organic compounds [9] contained in the plume. Some preliminary results of the joint project, which were presented on the conference 'Biomedical Optics Europe '93' in September 1993 in Budapest are summarized in the following [8–19]:

(a) Laser plume contains by order of magnitude: steam 70%, CO_2 13%, aerosol mass 13%, CO, HCN, NH_3, aldehyde, volatile organic compounds 4%.

(b) 90% of the aerosol particles are of sizes of 0.1 and 1.2 μm and therefore lung hazardous.

(c) The relation of CO and CO_2 production tends to higher amounts of CO the more carbonization occurs [10].

(d) The well-known plasma sparks which can be observed during the operation indicate increased production of CN molecules [13].

(e) The volatile organic compounds include by order of magnitude per 1 g of tissue ablation besides a large number of other pyrolysis products: benzene 40 μg; toluene 40 μg; styrene 20 μg; ethylbenzene 30 μg.

Among the pyrolysis products there is presumably a number of unknown substances [14]. Chemical analyses for their classification and identification are presently in progress.

References

1   Freitag L, Chapman GA, Sielczak M, Ahmed A, Russin D: Laser smoke effect on the bronchial system. Lasers Surg Med 1987;7:283–288.
2   Nezhat C, Winer KW, Nezhat F, Nezhat C, Forrest D, Reeves WG: Smoke from laser surgery: Is there a health hazard? Lasers Surg Med 1987;7:376–382.
3   Baggish MS, Elbakry M: The effects of laser smoke on the lungs of rats. Am J Obstet Gynecol 1987;156:1260–1265.
4   Walker NPJ, Matthews J, Newsom SWB: Possible hazards of lasers from irradiation with the carbon dioxide laser. Lasers Surg Med 1986;6:84–86.
5   Garden JM, O'Bannion MK, Shelnitz LS, Pinski KS, Bakus AD, Reichmann ME, Sundberg JP: Papillomavirus in the vapour of carbon dioxide laser-treated verrucae. JAMA 1988;259:1199–1202.
6   Hallmo P, Naess O: Laryngeal papillomatosis with human DNA contracted by a laser surgeon. Eur Arch Otolaryngol 1992;248:425–427.
7   Wöllmer W, Mihalache DL: Entwicklung eines Probenahme-Verfahrens für Schadstoff-Untersuchungen bei der Laserchirurgie; in Willital GM, Maragakis M, Lehmann RR (eds): Laser 92. Aachen, Verlag Shaker, 1992.

8   Albrecht H, Müller; State of the international project EU 642 STILMED – safety technology in Laser medicine; in van Gemert MJC, Steiner RW, Svaasand LO, Albrecht H (eds): Proceedings of 'Laser Interaction with Hard and Soft Tissue'. Bellingham, SPIE, 1994, vol 2077.

9   Weber L, Meier T: Review on toxicology of aerosols produced during medical laser treatment or electrosurgery; in van Gemert MJC, Steiner RW, Svaasand LO, Albrecht H (eds): Proceedings of 'Laser Interaction with Hard and Soft Tissue'. Bellingham, SPIE, 1994, vol 2077.

10 Weigmann HJ, Lademann J, Liebetruth J: Characterisation of laser tissue interaction by laser plume species; in van Gemert MJC, Steiner RW, Svaasand LO, Albrecht H (eds): Proceedings of 'Laser Interaction with Hard and Soft Tissue'. Bellingham, SPIE, 1994, vol 2077.

11 Albrecht H, Hagemann R, Wäsche W, Wagner G, Müller G: Volatile organic components in laser and electrosurgery plume; in van Gemert MJC, Steiner RW, Svaasand LO, Albrecht H (eds): Proceedings of 'Laser Interaction with Hard and Soft Tissue'. Bellingham, SPIE, 1994, vol 2077.

12 Meier T, Spleiss M, Treffler B, Weber L: Influence of laser parameters on by-products during laser treatment of biological tissues; in van Gemert MJC, Steiner RW, Svaasand LO, Albrecht H (eds): Proceedings of 'Laser Interaction with Hard and Soft Tissue'. Bellingham, SPIE, 1994, vol 2077.

13 Lademann J, Weigmann HJ: Laser spectroscopic detection of molecules and radicals during laser tissue interaction in laser plumes; in van Gemert MJC, Steiner RW, Svaasand LO, Albrecht H (eds): Proceedings of 'Laser Interaction with Hard and Soft Tissue'. Bellingham, SPIE, 1994, vol 2077.

14 Wöllmer W, Mihalache DL, Franke S, Francke W: Development and application of a minimized sampling procedure for access of early reaction products in laser plume analysis; in van Gemert MJC, Steiner RW, Svaasand LO, Albrecht H (eds): Proceedings of 'Laser Interaction with Hard and Soft Tissue'. Bellingham, SPIE, 1994, vol 2077.

15 Wäsche W, Wagner G, Albrecht H, Hagemann R, Müller G: Particle investigation as basis for toxicological assessment; in van Gemert MJC, Steiner RW, Svaasand LO, Albrecht H (eds): Proceedings of 'Laser Interaction with Hard and Soft Tissue'. Bellingham, SPIE, 1994, vol 2077.

16 Wagner G, Wäsche W, Albrecht H, Hagemann R, Müller G: Evaluation of laser plume distribution in operating theaters and potential risks; in van Gemert MJC, Steiner RW, Svaasand LO, Albrecht H (eds): Proceedings of 'Laser Interaction with Hard and Soft Tissue'. Bellingham, SPIE, 1994, vol 2077.

17 Meier T, Weber L, Grünvogel J, Treffler B: Visualisation of flow distribution at the evacuator nozzle; in van Gemert MJC, Steiner RW, Svaasand LO, Albrecht H (eds): Proceedings of 'Laser Interaction with Hard and Soft Tissue'. Bellingham, SPIE, 1994, vol 2077.

18 Wäsche W, Hagemann R, Albrecht H, Müller G: Efficiency of filters and evacuation systems; in van Gemert MJC, Steiner RW, Svaasand LO, Albrecht H (eds): Proceedings of 'Laser Interaction with Hard and Soft Tissue'. Bellingham, SPIE, 1994, vol 2077.

19 Liess HD, Lademann J: A new type of miniaturised drift sensor and its application in laser medicine; in van Gemert MJC, Steiner RW, Svaasand LO, Albrecht H (eds): Proceedings of 'Laser Interaction with Hard and Soft Tissue'. Bellingham, SPIE, 1994, vol 2077.

20 Wöllmer W, Koch U: Optimierung eines Mikrolaryngoskops für die Laser-Mikrolaryngoskopie. Zentralbl Hals Nasen Ohrenheilk Kopf Halschir 1994;145

Dr. Wolfgang Wöllmer, Universitäts-Hals-Nasen-Ohren-Klinik,
Universitätskrankenhaus Eppendorf, D–20246 Hamburg (Germany)

Rudert H, Werner JA (eds): Lasers in Otorhinolaryngology, and in Head and Neck Surgery.
Adv Otorhinolaryngol. Basel, Karger, 1995, vol 49, pp 23–26

Ophthalmological Risks and Hazards of Laser Use in the Head and Neck Region

Friederike U. Schmidt

Clinic for Ophthalmology, University of Kiel, Germany

The human eye is a highly specialised organ to process visible light but most susceptible to damage by extreme light intensities and wavelengths. All parts of the eye, as there are cornea, lens, vitreous cavity and retina, can be injured by visible light and infrared beams (400–1,400 nm). Near ultraviolet light (300–400 nm) is almost totally absorbed in the normal crystalline lens. The CO_2 laser, operating at 10.6 µm and the excimer laser operating at wavelengths below 300 nm are entirely absorbed at the corneal surface. The eye will be protected by lid and pupil reflexes and the tear film; however, laser radiation is too intensive and too fast for these mechanisms.

Therapeutic Laser Application to the Eye

Laser surgery has been used in ophthalmology since the invention of the instrument itself. Three different types are in use: coagulation, disruption and ablation [2–4, 7]. Coagulation is used in diabetic retinopathy and in the treatment of retinal holes with the argon laser.

Disruption is practiced by the Nd:YAG laser to cut the lens capsule in secondary cataract. The excimer laser has ablative properties in refractive surgery.

Ocular Injuries by Lasers of Different Wavelengths

Different laser light frequencies cause different eye injuries due to the absorption characteristics in water. CO_2 and excimer lasers can only injure the cornea, but argon, Nd:YAG, dye and copper vapor lasers can damage the retina. If the laser beam hits the fovea accidentally there will be a massive reduction in

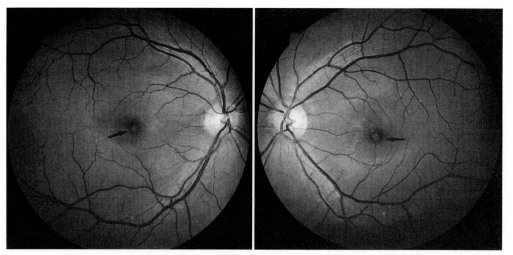

a   *b*

Fig. 1. a Right eye (retina) of a 32-year-old physicist with ruby laser injury in the macular area (arrow). *b* Left eye.

visual acuity. The practical importance of these injury patterns is illustrated by the following case report. A physicist was working with a ruby laser. After removing the protective eye glasses he touched the laser trigger by accident and hit both of his eyes in the central area (fig. 1a, b). His visual acuity decreased to 0.3 on both eyes. Cornea and lens can be damaged by laser beams absorbed by these ocular structures. This is the case for instance in CO_2 laser beams. The high metabolic rate of the cornea permits total epithelial repair when the epithelium alone is damaged superficially. A corneal scar can result if injury occurs in the deeper stromal layers of the cornea with higher laser intensities.

Only the wavelength regions UV-A and UV-B between 295 and 320 nm and IR-A and IR-B between 1 and 2 µm will preferentially cause injury to the crystalline lens. This accounts for Nd:YAG, copper vapor, argon and dye lasers (table 1). However, damage to other anatomic areas of the eye, especially the retina, may also occur.

Protective Measures

Eye protectors are the most important measures to prevent ocular injury [1, 5, 6]. Especially laser surgeons who work with Nd:YAG and copper vapor lasers (potentially hazardous for the retina) must wear suitable filter lenses. Specialized eye protection is now available for all types of lasers.

Table 1. Laser-specific eye injury patterns

	Wave-lengths, nm	Cor-nea	Lens	Vitre-ous	Retina
CO_2	10,600	X			
Excimer	193	X			
Nd:YAG	1,064	X	X	X	XX
Argon	488–514	X	X	X	X
Dye	500–800	X	X	X	X
Copper vapor	511–578	X	X	X	XX

Of the persons present in the operating room, the laser surgeon usually is least endangered since he is protected by the optical system delivering the laser light. If the laser surgeon operates by hand, he himself and every other person is potentially in danger. If the foot switch is pressed accidentally, injury can occur by direct and indirect (reflected) laser beams. The ophthalmic surgeon is protected by the slit lamp; the ENT surgeon by the operation microscope. In the latter case the distance between laser and patient is larger and can lead to accidental reflection.

It is extremely important to realize that normal glasses and sun glasses are by no means sufficient to prevent ocular laser damage. They do not possess special filters adapted to the wavelengths of the laser in use. Of course, the patient operated on must be included in the protective strategies. Normally, he should be given the same protective eye wear as the medical personnel. Periorbital laser use necessitates coverage of the eyelids with metallic foils. Laser application directly to the eyelids is possible with protective metal eye shields placed directly onto the bulbus. These commercially available protective devices are unnecessary, however, in the special case of the water-absorbed CO_2 laser. For microlaryngoscopy the eyes and face of the patient must simply be covered by wet gauze and clothes.

Every surgeon using medical lasers has to be knowledgeable about safety precautions and aware of frequency specific damages. It is his responsibility not only that all persons present in the operating theater including the patient are provided with the necessary safety gear, but also to prevent all avoidable deflection and reflection of the laser beam.

References

1   Eriksen P, Galoff PK: Measurements of laser eye protective filters. Health Phys 1989;56: 741–742.
2   L'Esperance FA Jr: Ophthalmic Lasers. St. Louis, Mosby, 1989, vol II.
3   Fankhauser F, Henchoz P-D, Kwasniewska E, van der Zypen E, England C, Rol P, Niederer P, Dürr U, Beck D: Chirurgie mit dem Laserskalpell. Physikalische Grundlagen und klinische Wirksamkeit. Klin Monatsbl Augenheilk 1993;203:436–443.
4   Kampik A (Hrsg): Laser-Jahrbuch der Augenheilkunde. Zülpich, Biermann Verlag, 1992.
5   Sliney DH, Le Boclott: Laser eye protectors. J Laser Appl 1990;2:9–13.
6   Sliney DH, Trokel SL: Medical Lasers and Their Safe Use. New York, Springer, 1993.
7   Wollensak J (Hrsg): Laser in der Ophthalmologie. Stuttgart, Enke Verlag, 1988.

Friederike U. Schmidt, MD, Clinic for Ophthalmology, University of Kiel,
Hegewischstrasse 2, D–24105 Kiel (Germany)

Rudert H, Werner JA (eds): Lasers in Otorhinolaryngology, and in Head and Neck Surgery.
Adv Otorhinolaryngol. Basel, Karger, 1995, vol 49, pp 27–30

Laser Delivery Systems and Laser Instruments in Otorhinolaryngology

Jochen A. Werner, Burkard M. Lippert, Matthias C. Heissenberg, Heinrich Rudert

Department of Otorhinolaryngology, Head and Neck Surgery,
University of Kiel, Germany

Because of the anatomic modalities laser applications in otorhinolaryngology have to fulfil particular requirements. The selection of laser delivery systems and laser instruments are determined by the type and location of the disease to be treated. In this medical speciality, the CO_2 laser is the most important applicable laser delivery system. In comparison to its medical use, Nd:YAG laser is distinctively more limited. The therapeutical margin of further laser delivery systems besides the two mentioned, is even narrower. Therefore, clinical applications and instruments for CO_2 laser and Nd:YAG laser will be emphasized in the following.

Meanwhile quite a number of corporations offer CO_2 and Nd:YAG laser delivery systems. The differences between the systems concern mainly working modes and power output parameters. The dependence of working modes and tissue effects was already illustrated by Lippert and co-workers in the first article of this book. Basically, tissue effects caused by the Nd:YAG laser are comparable to those caused by the CO_2 laser. In the following, we want to point out that the tissue effects of irradiated areas are mainly related to laser power density rather than to individual power parameters of different laser systems.

CO$_2$ Laser

Because of its small penetration depth the CO_2 laser's beam is mainly used as a cutting device rather than for vaporization and almost never for coagulation. In otorhinolaryngology, laser applications are almost exclusively performed using an operating microscope. The working distance for endola-

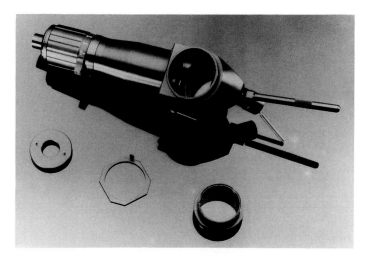

Fig. 1. Modern micromanipulator for CO_2 laser surgery. Reduction of laser energy output is achieved by diminishing the laser beam (711 Acuspot™, Sharplan, London).

ryngeal laser surgery is 400 mm. Most of the commercially available micromanipulators can focus the laser beam down to 0.6–0.8 mm in diameter. The latest development of new micromanipulators (for instance 711 Acuspot™, Sharplan, London; fig. 1) allow a focus reduction of 0.25 mm at 400 mm working distance. The effect of such a small beam diameter is obvious if one recalls that laser light related tissue effects are determined by laser power output, irradiated area and time of exposure.

We could demonstrate in morphological and clinical evaluations that identical laser energy densities did not cause the same tissue effects if the parameters laser power and laser radiated area varied. The use of increased power and of wider focus diameter (0.6–0.8 mm) caused a larger zone with carbonization and necrosis, if compared to power and focus reduced (0.25 mm) working mode with the same laser energy density used, respectively. The significantly higher amount of heat and its conductance in a high-power working mode results in more thermic damage of healthy tissue. Additionally, intraoperative bleeding increased by uncontrollable tissue rupture. Besides, the important differentiation of malignant tumor and healthy tissue under the operating microscope during a laser surgical resection of the tumor is much more difficult in the more power intense working mode than in the focus and power reduced mode [1].

The clinical use of focus and power reduced working mode will improve laser surgical cut and preparation qualities that way that limited carcinomas

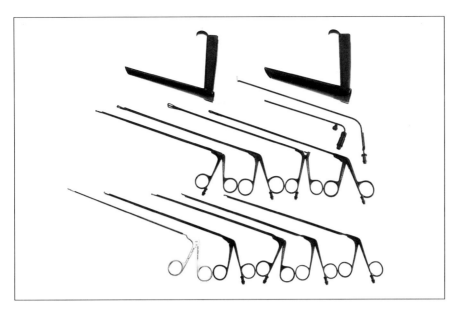

Fig. 2. Microsurgical instruments with suction channels for endolaryngeal CO_2 laser surgery (Storz, Tuttlingen).

can be removed more precisely than by using a high power mode. With this approach more healthy tissue can remain. The significance of laser-irradiated areas, and laser beam diameter for energy density results from the fact that laser energy increases four times if the beam diameter is halved, in contrast to reduction of the laser energy to 25% of its initial value if the focus diameter is doubled. A fact that justifies the use of new micromanipulators with reduction of laser beam diameter to less than 0.3 mm.

Since we have already published a report about the instruments we use for transoral laser surgery [2], only the most important aspects will be summarized in the following. We use Kleinsasser's laryngoscope [3] modified by Rudert [2] or the laryngoscope published by Weerda and Pedersen [4]. It is important to use laryngoscopes with additional suction channels. Microsurgical instruments are also provided with suction channels (fig. 2). Bleeding is stopped by electrocoagulation with an isolated suction tube, more intense bleeding by an isolated small forceps. The concern about the safety from the anesthesiological point of view and its avoidance by using special endotracheal tubes were already discussed in the preceding article by Jeckström and coworkers and previous publications by this group [5, 6].

Nd:YAG Laser

Nd:YAG laser is transmitted by a flexible fibreoptic light conductor that makes application in difficultly accessible areas possible. Special instruments for guidance of the flexible light conductor were developed like the laser rhinoscope, laser esophagoscope and laser bronchoscope.

In otorhinolaryngology, laser applications do not require more than 40 W. Most cases of Nd:YAG laser light applications are without contact. The light conductor is guided by hand. Special hand applicators with flexible tips allow the use in the nasopharynx and the maxillary sinuses. For precise applications and increased laser energy density at the tissue level, contact tips are available. The laser rhinoscope [7] has three service channels: one for exchangeable optical devices, a second for suction and a third for flexible light conductors for laser light transmission. Combined use of an angled optical device and a flexible light conductor laser light can be applied in even difficultly accessible areas and placed precisely under visual control.

References

1   Rudert H, Werner JA: Endoskopische Teilresektion mit dem CO_2-Laser bei Larynxkarzinomen. I. Resektionstechniken. Laryngo Rhino Otol 1994;73:71–77.
2   Rudert H: Instrumentarium für die CO2-Laser-Chirurgie. HNO 1989;37:76–77.
3   Kleinsasser O: Weitere technische Entwicklung und erste Ergebnisse der 'endolaryngealen Mikrochirurgie'. Z Laryngol Rhinol 1965;44:711–727.
4   Weerda H, Pedersen W: Ein neues Spreizlaryngoskop für die endolaryngeale Diagnostik und Mikrochirurgie. HNO 1981;29:58–63.
5   Werner JA, Schade W, Jeckström W, Lippert BM, Godbersen GS, Helbig V, Rudert H: Comparison of endotracheal tube safety during carbon dioxide laser surgery: an experimental study. Laser Med Surg 1990;6:184–189, 197.
6   Jeckström W, Wawersik J, Werner JA: Narkosetechnik bei laserchirurgischen Eingriffen im Kehlkopfbereich. HNO 1992;40:28–32.
7   Werner JA, Rudert H: Der Einsatz des Nd:YAG-Lasers in der Hals-, Nasen-, Ohrenheilkunde. HNO 1992;40:248–258.

Priv.-Doz. Dr. Jochen A. Werner, Department of Otorhinolaryngology, Head and Neck Surgery, University of Kiel, Arnold-Heller-Strasse 14, D–24105 Kiel (Germany)

Rudert H, Werner JA (eds): Lasers in Otorhinolaryngology, and in Head and Neck Surgery.
Adv Otorhinolaryngol. Basel, Karger, 1995, vol 49, pp 31–35

....

Mechanisms of Phototoxic Effects in Photodynamic Therapy

Thomas P.U. Wustrow

Department of Otorhinolaryngology, Head and Neck Surgery,
Ludwig-Maximilians-University, Munich, Germany

Photodynamic therapy (PDT) tries to reach an additional place as a further oncologic treatment modality. In order to determine the exact indications in appropriate controlled and randomized studies, the individual determinants of the photodynamic effects have to be considered [1]. Several effects generating the tumor cell destruction are responsible for the photodynamic effect: (1) the photosensitizer with its individual biologic properties; (2) the application of the photosensitizer with its destruction in tissues and cells; (3) the light quality and distribution in the tissue; (4) the acute and late phototoxic effects [2].

Photosensitizers

There is an enormous variability in characteristics for various photosensitizers. Thus, there is a strong difference in the time interval between intravenous application and maximal tissue concentration. Furthermore, the retention and binding of the photosensitizer differ significantly resulting in the variable appearance of the skin photosensitization. According to the chemical characteristics of the photosensitizer, the effects are dependent on the photosensitizer localization. Today a number of photosensitizers are in use or in research (table 1).

The dye localization is, however, also dependent on the chemical composition of the dye. Lipophilic anionic dyes attach more to membrane structures like the plasma membrane, mitochondrial membrane, the endoplasmic reticulum membrane or even the nuclear membrane [3]. Increased damage of tumor cells with high mitochondrial content [4] has been described in head and neck

Table 1. Photosensitizers

AlPcSn	sulfonated chloroaluminum phthalocyanine
P II	photofrin II (mixture of lipophilic materials)
SnET2	metallopurpurin
NPe6	mono-L-aspartyl chlorin e6
bChla	bacteriochlorophyll a
PcS	sulfonated phthalocyanines
BPD-MA	benzoporphyrin derivative
TPPS$_4$	hydrophilic tetrasulfonated tetraphenylporphines
TPPS$_1$	lipophilic sulfonated derivative of tetraphenylporphines
ALA	5-aminolevulinic acid
Zupc	Zn-phthalocyanine
isoBoSiNc	Si-naphthalocyanine
EDKC	cyanine dye
HPD	hematoporphyrinderivative

cancer cell lines and mitochondrial targeting seems to be a major action in photosensitization [5]. Hydrophilic dyes, on the other hand, bind to lysosomes [6] whereas cationic dyes are predominantly localized on the mitrochondria due to the electrical potential gradients. These different actions are dependent on the chemical compositions of each dye and have to be considered when different dyes are used. Besides the uptake, enormous differences exist for each of the photosensitizers regarding their clearance abilities, which are due to different distributions of the photosensitizers among different tumor compartments and to different sensitivity of normal and tumor-derived cells [7]. Moreover, the degree of sulfonation results in a variable photosensitization [8].

In a number of papers, and mostly clinically oriented papers, it is stated that there is a selective destruction of tumor cells by HPD. A question arises if sensitizers do or do not accumulate selectively in neoplastic tissues. Most evidence arises that the accumulation is not selective in neoplastic tissues due to: (1) likely differential sensitizer concentrations between tumor and the surrounding normal tissues; (2) only a very limited binding of the photosensitizer to the tumor cells itself; (3) a pooling of sensitizers in tumors due to a leaky tumor vasculature and poor lymphatic drainage of the tumor; (4) the aggregation, charge distribution and polarity properties of the photosensitizers [9], and (5) an unspecific uptake via the lipoprotein pathway especially the LDL receptor-mediated endocytosis.

There is considerable variation between the different photosensitizers due to the time interval between administration and peak sensitizer tissue levels and sensitizer retention. Both mechanisms are important for the effects of PDT.

Light Delivery

The light influence decreases exponentially with the distance. The light effects are influenced: (1) by optical absorption, caused by endogenous chromophores; (2) by optical scattering within the tissue, and (3) self-shielding which means an absorption of light by the photosensitizer itself.

Most important is the photobleaching which is a photodestruction of the photosensitizer during light exposure [10].

Photodynamic Effects

The photodynamic effects are dependent on the photosensitizer (today mostly photofrin II is used), the light of appropriate wavelength (mostly used 630 nm) and a sufficient oxygen supply. The photocytotoxicity in PDT occurs in a reaction where singlet oxygen is generated [11]. This damages cell structures like the plasma membranes, cytoplasmatic organelles, enyzmes or nuclear structures. Furthermore, the generation of singlet oxygen has a direct effect on the microcirculation resulting in cell swelling and interstitial fluid accumulation.

Acute Effects of PDT

The acute effects of PDT are, on the one hand, cellular and, on the other, vascular. As cellular effects, the photoperoxidation of membrane cholesterol and other unsaturated phospholipids are considered [12, 13]. Thus, the membrane permeability is increased and this results in a loss of fluidity. Furthermore, there is a cross-linking of aminolipids and polypeptides and an inactivation of membrane-associated enzymes and receptors. In addition, mitrochondrial enzymes and functions are significantly inhibited [4, 5]. The second main cellular effect is DNA damage [14].

Only few publications have appeared on the acute cellular effects caused by the release of inflammatory and immune mediators [15, 16]. Most important are the influences of the arachnoic acid system [17] as well as the histamine release [18] resulting in vasoactive contractions. Moreover, procoagulant factor VIII and TNF-α [19] are released which results again in further vascular contractions and reduced blood flow.

Besides the cellular effects vascular effects are most important in the acute effects of PDT [20]. As already mentioned by release of certain cytokines, especially of TNF-α, IL-1β and IL-2 [21], vascular effects as well as inflammatory responses are induced. Up to now it is not known how much an increased platelet aggregation is stimulated by PDT [22]. Disturbances of the vascular wall resulting in a further release of mediators are well established. Most important, however, is the level of the circulating photosensitizer which influences directly the needed light dosage. Those tumors with reduced blood flow velocity or increased compartments of hypoxic tumor cell fractions which both protect the tumor cells from further PDT damage due to hypoxia or insufficient oxygen supply, have been considered unfavorable [23, 24].

Late Effects of PDT

The prolonged cutaneous photosensitivity for which the patient has to avoid any natural light exposure for about 2 months, as in Photofrin II [25], is most disturbing for the patients. A number of agents have been used like diuretics, metabolic modifiers or WR 2721 for reducing the cutaneous photosensitivity but this was only mildly successful [26, 27]. Depending on the light dosage and the characteristics of the photosensitizer, the nature of the skin healing and the mutagenic or carcinogenic events which have to be analyzed for each photosensitizer are influenced [28].

Conclusion

The complex nature of the cellular and vascular responses to PDT treatment has not yet been fully understood. Ongoing studies try to clarify many of the questions which remain open and have to be answered before further extensive clinical trials are initiated and before PDT will gain its steady place as a further modality in cancer treatment.

References

1   Henderson BW, Dougherty TJ: How does photodynamic therapy work? Photochem Photobiol 1992;55:145–157.
2   Musser DA, Wagner JF, Datta-Gupta N: The interaction of tumor localizing porphyrins with collagen and elastin. Res Commun Chem Pathol Pharmacol 1982;36:251–259.
3   Moan JK, Berg EK van, Western A, Malik Z, Ruck A, Schneckenburger H: Intracellular localization of photosensitizers, in Bock G (ed): Photosensitizing Compounds: Their Chemistry, Biology and Clinical Use. Chichester, Wiley, 1989, pp 95–107.
4   Schneckenburger H, Wustrow TPU: Intracellular fluorescence of photosensitizing porphyrins at different concentrations of mitochondria. Photochem Photobiol 1988;47:471–473.
5   Salet C, Moreno G: New trends in photobiology. Photosensitization of mitochondria. Molecular and cellular aspects. J Photochem Photobiol 1990;5:133–150.
6   Zdolsek JM, Olsson GM, Brunk UT: Photooxidative damage to lysosomes of cultured macrophages by acridine orange. Photochem Photobiol 1990;51:67–76.

7   Mathews EK, Cui ZJ: Photodynamic action of sulphonated aluminium phthalocyanine (SALPC) on normal and carcinoma cells of the rat exocrine pancreas. 3rd Biennial-Meet Int Photodynamic Assoc, Buffalo, N. Y., July 1990, abstr VI/7.

8   Brasseur N, Ali H, Langlois R, van Lier JE: Biological activities of phthalocyanines. IX. Photo-sensitization of V-79 Chinese hamster cells and EMT-6 mouse mammary tumor by selectively sulfonated zinc phthalocyanines. Photochem Photobiol 1988;47:705–711.

9   Kongshaug M, Moan J, Brown SB: The distribution of porphyrins with different tumor localising ability among human plasma proteins. Br J Cancer 1989;59:184–188.

10   Potter WR: The theory of PDT dosimetry: Consequences of photodestruction of sensitizer. Photochem Photobiol 1987;46:97–101.

11   Foote CS: Chemical mechanisms of photodynamic action. Proc SPIE Institute 'Advanced Optical Technologies on Photodynamic Therapy', IS 6 1990, pp 115–126.

12   Girotti AW: Photodynamic lipid peroxidation in biological systems. Photochem Photobiol 1990;51:497–509.

13   Thomas JP, Girotti AW: Role of lipid peroxidation in hematoporphyrin derivative-sensitized photo-killing of tumor cells: Protective effects of glutathione peroxidase. Cancer Res 1989;49:1682–1686.

14   Ramakrishnan N, Oleinick NL, Clay ME, Horng MF, Antunez AR, Evans HH: DNA lesions and DNA degradation in mouse lymphoma L5178Y cells after photodynamic treatment sensitized by chloroaluminum phthalocyanine. Photochem Photobiol 1989;50:373–378.

15   Ferrario A, Gomer CJ: Systemic toxicity in mice induced by localized porphyrin photodynamic therapy. Cancer Res 1990;50:539–543.

16   Fingar VH, Wieman TJ, Doak KW: Role of thromboxane and prostacyclin release on photodynamic therapy-induced tumor destruction. Cancer Res 1990;50:2599–2603.

17   Henderson BW, Donovan JM: Release of prostaglandin E$_2$ from cells by photodynamic treatment in vitro. Cancer Res 1989;49:6896–6900.

18   Kerdel FA, Soter NA, Lim HW: In vivo mediator release and degranulation of mast cells in hematoporphyrin derivative-induced phototoxicity in mice. J Invest Dermatol 1987;88:277–280.

19   Evans S, Matthews W, Perry R, Fraker D, Norton J, Pass HI: Effect of photodynamic therapy on tumor necrosis factor production by murine macrophages. J Natl Cancer Inst 1990;82:34–39.

20   Feyh J, Goetz A, Conzen P, Brendel W: Microcirculatory effects of photoradiation therapy (PRT) with hematoporphyrin derivative. Int J Microcirc 1987;6:91.

21   Nseyo UO, Whalen R, Duncan MR, Berman B, Lundahl SL: Urinary cytokines following photodynamic therapy for bladder cancer: A preliminary report. Urology 1990;36:167–171.

22   Henderson BW, Sweeney J, Gessner T: Endothelial cell production of physiologic mediators in response to PDT in vitro and effects on platelet function. Photochem Photobiol 1991;53:96.

23   Reed MWR, Miller FN, Wieman TJ, Tseng MT, Pietsch CG: The effect of photodynamic therapy on the microcirculation. J Surg Res 1988;45:452–459.

24   Henderson BW, Fingar VH: Oxygen limitation of direct tumor cell killing during photodynamic treatment. Photochem Photobiol 1989;49:299–304.

25   Dougherty TJ, Cooper MT, Mang TS: Cutaneous phototoxic occurrences in patients receiving Photofrin. Lasers Surg Med 1990;10:485–488.

26   Manyak MJ, Smith PD, Harrington FS, Steinbert SM, Glatstein E, Russo A: Protection against dihematoporphyrin ether sensitively. Photochem Photobiol 1988;47:823–830.

27   Bellnier DA, Dougherty TA: Protection of murine skin and transplantable tumor against Photofrin II mediated photodynamic sensitization with WR-2721. J Photochem Photobiol 1989;4:219–225.

28   Evans HH, Rerko RM, Mencl J, Clay ME, Antunez AR, Oleinick NL: Cytotoxic and mutagenic effects of the photodynamic action of chloroaluminum phthalocyanine and visible light in L5178Y cells. Photochem Photobiol 1989;49:43–47.

Prof. Dr. Thomas P. U. Wustrow, Department of Otorhinolaryngology, Head and Neck Surgery, Ludwig-Maximilians-University, Marchioninistrasse 15, D–81377 München (Germany)

Rudert H, Werner JA (eds): Lasers in Otorhinolaryngology, and in Head and Neck Surgery.
Adv Otorhinolaryngol. Basel, Karger, 1995, vol 49, pp 36–38

....

Experimental Photodynamic Therapy of the Larynx Using 5-Aminolaevulinic Acid

Detlef Kleemann [a,b], *Alexander J. MacRobert* [a], *Thomas Mentzel* [c],
Stephen G. Brown [a,1]

[a] National Medical Laser Centre, Department of Surgery, University College,
London, UK;
[b] ENT Clinic 'Otto Körner', University of Rostock, Germany;
[c] St. Thomas' Hospital London, Soft Tissue Tumour Unit, UK

Photodynamic therapy (PDT) of head and neck tumours has attracted increasing attention over the last 10 years, as shown by more than 30 recent clinical publications. However, despite the inherent suitability of PDT for laryngeal tumours, only a few studies have been performed on this organ to date. The greater accessibility for light irradiation to other parts of the head and neck region such as the oral cavity may account partly for this comparative neglect. Nevertheless, PDT is promising as a function preserving treatment, especially for small laryngeal malignancies, laryngeal papillomatosis and precancerous lesions of the larynx. Haematoporphyrin derivative (HpD) and its purified versions remain the most widely used clinical photosensitizers. Although good clinical results using these sensitizers have been reported, they have certain disadvantages, particularly the long-lasting skin photosensitivity, which has prompted an active search for new photosensitizers with more suitable properties.

There has been much recent interest in the endogeneous protoporphyrin IX (PP IX) photosensitization induced by administration of exogeneous 5-aminolaevulinic acid (ALA). Photodynamic effects have been produced both in vitro and in vivo after ALA application and subsequent exposure to red light at 630 nm [1, 2]. Compared with HpD, the great advantage of ALA is the

[1] D. Kleemann and Th. Mentzel were funded by the German Academic Exchange Service (DAAD). We are grateful for support from The Imperial Cancer Research Fund and DUSA Inc.

short duration of sensitization of most tissues. More recently, several experimental and clinical studies using ALA have been reported showing that, unlike other currently available photosensitizers, it can be given either topically or systematically (orally or intravenously) [3–5].

We have examined the distribution of ALA induced PP IX fluorescence in the tissues of the normal rabbit larynx at different time points after administration of various doses (20, 100 and 200 mg/kg body weight) of ALA. Quantitative fluorescence imaging of frozen larynx sections was carried out with a fluorescence microscope, attached to a CCD (charge-coupled device) camera system.

With the dose of 200 mg/kg ALA, the fluorescence signal in the mucosa rose rapidly to a peak at 4 h whilst the integrated signal in the other layers rose more slowly. The submucosa (except the submucosal glands) as well as the muscle exhibited relatively little fluorescence. The ratio between mucosa and both of these tissues reached approximately 7:1 at the peak time of 4 h. In contrast, the signal in cartilage increased at a markedly slower rate reaching a much later maximum around 48 h. There was no detectable fluorescence in any tissue after 1 week. The peak fluorescence in mucosa was achieved earlier with lower doses of ALA and declined more rapidly. Peak levels after 100 mg/kg were comparable after 200 mg/kg, with the allowance for experimental error, but were attained 1 h earlier.

PDT necrosis of squamous cell carcinomas, the most common tumour of the larynx is well documented. However, for PDT to be of clinical value it is essential for the nature of the damage and subsequent recovery of the adjacent normal tissues to be fully understood. This is of particular importance in an organ such as the larynx whose function is very sensitive to small changes in its component tissues. The aim of this work therefore was to assess the damage and subsequent healing of normal laryngeal tissues following PDT treatment. So we treated rabbits with IV ALA injections and exposed the vocal cord area via tracheotomy to laser light at 630 nm (fibre output 100 mW, total light dose 100 J/cm^2) and followed up the animals to 6 weeks after the procedure.

Untreated animals (sensitizer only) and those with just a tracheotomy showed no histological changes, although the group of animals exposed to laser light only did show some mild reactive changes. Using increasing amounts of ALA (20, 100 and 200 mg/kg), increasing degrees of necrosis, inflammatory infiltration, and fibrosis were observed in all regions studied after laser irradiation. With 200 mg/kg and laser irradiation at 4 h, necrosis and fibrosis of deep striated muscle were clearly evident. In contrast, with 100 mg/kg and laser treatment at 3 h, the zone of necrosis was confined to the mucosal layer and superficial seromucous glands, with no evident necrosis of cartilage or muscle. Long-term results (6 weeks) demonstrated re-epithelization of the true and false vocal cords and only moderate subepithelial fibrosis in the group sensitised with 100 mg/kg ALA. With the 200 mg/kg, 10 days after the treatment the mucosa was already regenerating, but at 6 weeks, there was continuous band-like intramuscular fibrosis with no indication of muscle or cartilage regeneration.

We conclude that using ALA, it may be possible to treat mucosal lesions of the larynx safety as long as the dose is not excessive. The choice of the laser treatment time point after sensitization may also be critical. Some questions remain to be proven in clinical studies on laryngeal tumours.

References

1 Malik Z, Lugaci H: Destruction of erythroleucaemic cells by photoactivation of endogenous porphyrins. Br J Cancer 1987;56:589–595.
2 Divaris DSG, Kennedy JC, Pottier RH: Phototoxic damage to sebaceous glands and hair follicels of mice after systemic administration of 5-aminolaevulinic acid correlates with localized protoporphyrin IX fluorescence. Am J Pathol 1990;136:891–897.
3 Kennedy JC, Pottier RH: Endogenous protoporphyrin IX, a clinically useful photosensitizer for photodynamic therapy. J Photochem Photobiol [B] 1992;14:275–292.
4 Loh CS, MacRobert AJ, Bedwell J, Regula J, Krasner N, Bown SG: Oral versus intravenous administration of 5-aminolaevulinic acid for photodynamic therapy. Br J Cancer 1993;68:41–51.
5 Grant WE, Hopper C, Speight P, Bown SG: Photodynamic therapy of oral cancer: Photosensitisation with systemic aminolaevulinic acid. Lancet 1993;342:147.

Dr. med. D. Kleemann, Klinik und Poliklinik für Hals-Nasen-Ohren-Krankheiten
'Otto Körner', Universität Rostock, Doberaner Strasse 137–139,
D–18057 Rostock (Germany)

Rudert H, Werner JA (eds): Lasers in Otorhinolaryngology, and in Head and Neck Surgery.
Adv Otorhinolaryngol. Basel, Karger, 1995, vol 49, pp 39–43

Experimental Studies on the Phototoxic Effect of Cytostatic Agents

Results and Outlook

B.M. Lippert [a], *W. Schade* [b], *S. Gottschlich* [a], *J.A. Werner* [a]

[a] Department of Otorhinolaryngology, Head and Neck Surgery
  (Chairman: Prof. *H. Rudert*), and
[b] Institute for Experimental Physics (Chairman: Prof. *A. Piel*),
  University of Kiel, Germany

Over the past few years, photodynamic therapy (PDT) has developed into an effective therapeutic method for small superficial malignant tumors and has been applied highly successfully in treating various malignant tumors [4, 6]. Usually, hematoporphyrin derivates (HPD) are used as photosensitizers. PDT with HPD has several disadvantages limiting its clinical use. The main problem is the phototoxicity to the skin [17]. Other disadvantages are that HPD has no significant tumor selectivity [3] and that the penetration depth of the laser light is rather small so that only superficial tumors can be treated successfully [11, 20].

Several modifications and clinical trials have been published in recent years with the intent to increase the effectivity of PDT [3, 11, 16]. One possibility to increase the effect of PDT is the combination with chemotherapy. The basic idea behind a combination therapy with cytostatic drugs is to utilize the cytostatic properties of these agents in addition to the photodynamic effect and to thus enhance the overall effect on the tumor [5, 15]. Because of their photochemical properties, anthracyclin derivatives seem to be especially suited for photodynamic therapy. Besides their direct effect on the DNA, these substances also release highly reactive radicals without requiring any additional laser light irradiation. These radicals can react with the cell organelles and the cell membranes [1, 10, 18].

Material and Methods

Cell Cultivation

For all experiments, we used a recloned squamous cell carcinoma line of the oral cavity, which was cultivated as previously reported [8].

Photosensitizers and Light Source

The anthracyclin derivatives adriamycin, daunomycin and epirubicin served as photosensitizers (Farmitalia Carlo Erba, Italy). Solutions of different concentrations were prepared (0.1–10 µg/ml). We used an argon laser (wavelength 488/514 nm) at the Kiel University Institute of Experimental Physics for our experiments.

Photosensitization and Laser Irradiation

A modified experimental model developed by Wustrow et al. [20] was used for photosensitization and irradiation of the tumor cells, as previously reported [12]. 2×10^5/ml cells were irradiated with laser light at wavelengths of 488/514 nm. Maximum radiant energy amounted to 5 J/cm^2. After 24 and 48 h live and destroyed cells were distinguished from each other in a vitality test using 0.5% trypan blue. The cells were compared with a control group that had not been treated.

Results

Cell Growth without PDT

Daunomycin could not reduce the cell growth in the tested concentrations. Therefore, it was not used for the following laser light irradiation. Compared to the control group, cell growth was suppressed by only 15–20% after exposure to adriamycin concentrations ranging from 1 to 4 µg/ml. With adriamycin concentrations of 5 µg/ml and more, however, a pronounced cytostatic effect could be observed since the reduction in growth amounted to more than 50%. Cell growth was stopped almost completely at concentrations of 9 µg/ml and more. Depending on the concentration, cell growth was also reduced following epirubicin incubation. The cytostatic effect was slightly more pronounced than with adriamycin (fig. 1).

Cell Growth with PDT

A comparison of the cytostatic effect of adriamycin with or without laser light irradiation revealed a distinct photodynamic effect. 75–80% of the cells survived if only the cytotoxic agent with concentrations of 1–3 µg/ml was administered. With PDT the number increased to more than 50%. Virtually all cells were destroyed at concentrations of 3 µg/ml or more. The photodynamic effect of epirubicin was almost just as pronounced. Compared to adriamycin, however, the overall lethal action of epirubicin was slightly more effective due to the stronger cytostatic effect (fig. 2).

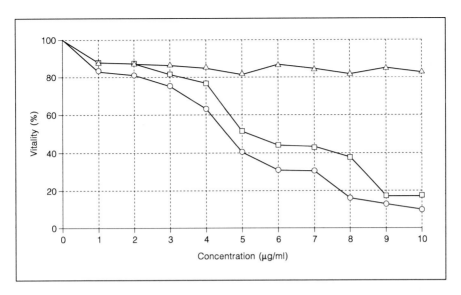

Fig. 1. Cell survival after incubation with adriamycin (□), daunomycin (△) and epirubicin (○).

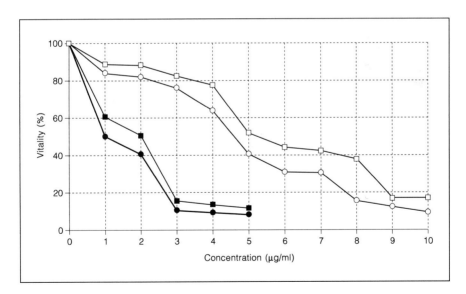

Fig. 2. Cell survival after adriamycin incubation alone (□) and with laser irradiation (■) and after epirubicin incubation alone (○) and with laser irradiation (●).

Discussion

Photodynamic therapy done with hematoporphyrin derivatives is established as an independent therapeutic procedure and was used successfully in treating various cases of superficial malignant growth [7, 17, 19]. Only few studies on the interaction between photodynamic therapy and cytostatic agents have been published [2, 9, 13]. Among many different cytostatic agents the anthracyclin derivatives adriamycin and epirubicin seem to be especially suited for a synergic therapy [2, 5]. Our own studies, which are in agreement with those of other authors, showed that the cytostatic drugs cisplatin, 5-fluorouracil and methotrexate, which are very effective in treating squamous cell carcinoma, were unsuited for photodynamic therapy because of their unfavorable absorption capacities [2, 9, 13].

In our experiments we could demonstrate that adriamycin and epirubicin do not only possess cytostatic efficacy but also a marked photodynamic effect. Similar to the action of hematoporphyrin derivatives, both substances concentrate in mitochondria of fast-proliferating cells [14] and destroy the cells by releasing highly toxic oxygen radicals [1]. In addition to the cytostatic action of the anthracyclin derivatives, a photodynamic effect can be achieved by laser irradiation, which enhances the overall effect on the tumor without causing any additional side effects.

Outlook

PDT with HPD is useful in the treatment of small superficial malignancies. It is of no use in the therapy of large malignancies of the head and neck. Promising therapeutic modifications are clinical trials with new photosensitizers and the combination of PDT with chemotherapy. The combination or a preoperative adjuvant chemotherapy followed by tumor excision and intraoperative laser light irradiation of the tumor area and the excisional borders might successfully treat tumor residues of microscopic size. PDT might even contribute to the treatment of large malignancies as part of this combination therapy. This is especially true for the head and neck area where large tumors can often only be partially resected due to the anatomic situation.

References

1   Alegria AE, Riesz GR: Photochemistry of aqueous adriamycin and daunomycin. A spin trapping study with ^{17}O enriched oxygen and water. Photochem Photobiol 1988;48:147–152.
2   Cowled PA, Mackenzie L, Forbes IJ: Pharmacological modulation of photodynamic therapy with hematoporphyrin derivative and light. Cancer Res 1987;47:971–974.

3   Davis RK: Photodynamic therapy in otolaryngology-head and neck surgery. Otolaryng Clin North Am 1990;1:107–119.
4   Dougherty TJ, Lawrence G, Kaufman JH, Boyle D, Weishaupt KR, Goldfarb A: Photoradiation in the treatment of recurrent breast carcinoma. J Natl Cancer Inst 1979;62:231–237.
5   Edell ES, Cortese DA: Combined effects of hematoporphyrin derivative phototherapy and adriamycin in a murine tumor model. Lasers Surg Med 1988;8:413–417.
6   Edge CJ, Carruth AS: Photodynamic therapy and the treatment of head and neck cancer. Br J Oral Maxillofac Surg 1988;26:1–11.
7   Feyh J, Goetz AH, Martin F, Lumper W, Müller W, Brendel W, Kastenbauer E: Photodynamische Lasertumortherapie mit Hämatoporphyrin-Derivat (HpD) eines Spinozellulären Karzinomes der Ohrmuschel. Laryngo Rhino Otol 1989;68:563–565.
8   Görögh T, Eickbohm JE, Ewers R, Lippert BM, Holdener EE: Inhibited methionine incorporation in human squamuos carcinomas of the oral cavity as a measure for response to 5-fluorouacil. J Cancer Res Clin Oncol 1989;115:366–372.
9   Gossner L, Wittke H, Warzechna A, Ernst H, Sroka R, Hahn EG, Ell CH: Combination of chemotherapy and photodynamic therapy of human gastrointestinal tumor xenografts in nude mice; in Waidelich W, Waidelich R, Hofstetter A (ed): Laser in Medicine. Berlin, Springer, 1992, pp 141–148.
10 Gray PJ, Phillips DR: Ultraviolet photoirradiation of daunomycin and DNA-daunomycin complexes. Photochem Photobiol 1980;33:297–303.
11 Heinritz H, Benzel W, Sroka R, Iro H: Fluoreszenzdiagnostik und photodynamische Therapie von oberflächlichen Hauttumoren nach topischer Applikation von Delta-Aminolävulinsäure. Eur Arch Otorhinolaryngol 1993;(suppl II):171–172.
12 Lippert BM, Werner JA, Schade W, Rudert H: Zytostatika-induzierte Phototoxizität bei Plattenepithelkarzinomen – Erste erfolgversprechende Ergebnisse einer in-vitro-Untersuchung. Eur Arch Otorhinolaryngol 1991;(suppl II):76–77.
13 Liwei M, Zhonghe G, Chenggui L, Yanyong J: The synergistic killing effects of photodynamic therapy cooperated with mitomycin C on the human colon adenocarcinoma cells (LS174T) experimental study and clinical application. Lasermedizin 1990;0:5–8.
14 Samal AB, Frolov AA: An influence of adriamycin and light on Aggregation of human platelets; in Spinelli P, Dal Frank M, Marchesini R (cd): Photodynamic Therapy and Biomedical Lasers. Amsterdam, Excerpta Medica, 1992, pp 826–829.
15 Sanfilippo A, Schioppacassi G, Morvillo E, Ghione M: Photodynamic action of daunomycin. I. Effect on bacteriophage T2 and bacteria. G Microbiol 1968;16:49–54.
16 Schmidt S, Schultes B, Wagner U, Oehr P, Decleer W, Lubaschowski H, Biersack HJ, Krebs D: Photodynamic laser therapy of carcinomas-effects of five different photosensitizers in colony-forming assay. Arch Gynecol Obstet 1991;249:9–14.
17 Schweitzer VG: Photodynamic therapy for treatment of head and neck cancer. Otolaryngol Head Neck Surg 1990;102:225–232.
18 Verini MA, Casazza AM, Fioretti A, Rodenghi F, Ghione M: Photodynamic action of daunomycin. II. Effect on animal viruses. G Microbiol 1968;16:55–64.
19 Wenig BL, Kurtzman DM, Grosweiner LI, Mafee MF, Harris DM, Lobraico RV, Prycz RA, Appelbaum EL: Photodynamic therapy in the treatment of squamous cell carcinoma of the head and neck. Arch Otolaryngol Head Neck Surg 1990;116:1267–1270.
20 Wustrow TPU, Jocham D, Schramm A, Unsöld E: Photodynamische Zerstörung in vitro kultivierter Plattenepithelkarzinomzellen aus dem Kopf-Hals-Bereich. Laryngo Rhino Otol 1988; 67:532–538.

Dr. B.M. Lippert, Department of Otolaryngology, Head and Neck Surgery, University of Kiel, Arnold-Heller-Strasse 14, D–24105 Kiel (Germany)

Rudert H, Werner JA (eds): Lasers in Otorhinolaryngology, and in Head and Neck Surgery.
Adv Otorhinolaryngol. Basel, Karger, 1995, vol 49, pp 44–47

....

Meta-Tetrahydroxyphenylchlorin: A New Photosensitizer for Photodynamic Therapy of Head and Neck Tumors

H. Heinritz [a], *F. Waldfahrer* [a], *W. Benzel* [a], *R. Sroka* [b], *H. Iro* [a]

[a] Department of Otorhinolaryngology, University of Erlangen-Nürnberg, and
[b] GSF-Zentrales Laserlaboratorium, Neuherberg, Germany

For more than a decade, the hematoporphyrin derivative (HPD) has been almost solely used in photodynamic therapy. However, it is well known to have a number of disadvantages. First, it is a complex mixture of various porphyrin monomers, dimers and polymers, some of them obviously inactive in vivo [1]. Second, tissue penetration of light in the range able to activate photosensitizers increases with wavelength [2, 3], and, thus, for effective tumor damage, illumination should be at the longest wavelength that excites the sensitizer. For HPD (625–630 nm), this is a poorly effective excitation band. Other disadvantages relate to tissue selectivity of photosensitization. HPD sensitizes skin, so that patients must avoid strong light for at least 3 weeks up to several months after treatment. A partly purified preparation of HPD, said to be enriched in di-hematoporphyrin ether is available for clinical studies as Photofrin II® or Photosan III®. Even though it has advantages, there are no principle differences to HPD. It would be preferable to have photosensitizers that are pure materials and which are strongly activated by red light, preferably at the more penetrating wavelengths (above 630 nm). In the search for desirable photosensitizers, favored candidates are phthalocyanines [4, 5] and chlorins [6]. We have studied the photodynamic effect of meta-tetrahydroxyphenylchlorin (mTHPC) in comparison to Photosan III in a human squamous carcinoma cell line derived from the hypopharynx.

Material and Methods

Photosensitizers
Photosan III was obtained from Seehof Laboratories, Wesselburenerkoog (Germany). Scotia Pharmaceuticals Ltd., Guildford (UK) provided mTHPC.

Cell Culture
The experiments were performed with a human squamous carcinoma cell line derived form of the hypopharynx (FaDu, 7). Monolayer cultures were maintained at 37 °C and 5% of CO_2 in DME medium supplemented with 10% fetal calf serum, 50 µg/ml penicillin, 50 µg/ml streptomycin and 2.3 µg/ml amphotericin B (all obtained from Gibco). 24 h previous to application of a photosensitizer the cells were washed by centrifugation and 2×10^5 cells/ml in fresh DME medium were seeded into tissue culture flasks (Falcon Inc.). The cells were then incubated in the dark for either 24, 48 and 72 h containing Photosan III or mTHPC (0.1, 0.5, 1, 5 and 10 µg/ml). After viability testing (trypan blue method), the cells were again incubated with Photosan III (0.5 µg/ml) and mTHPC (0.5 µg/ml). Then the lids of each dish were removed and the cells were exposed to red light (630 and 650 nm). The delivered light doses ranged from 2 to 8 J/cm². The cells were then refed with DME medium and 3–5 h later the viability was assessed by the ability of cells to exclude trypan blue. Three dishes were treated at each dose point.

Light Source
An argon dye laser ('MDS 90', Aesculap-Meditec, Heroldsberg/Germany) was used as light source. Light was passed down a 0.5-mm fibre and interfaced with a microlens to broaden and even out the intensity of the delivered light. The light intensity (measured with power meter: Mod 212, Coherent Inc.) was 100 mW/cm², where thermal effects with red light are negligible. Excitation wavelengths were 630 nm for Photosan III and 650 nm for m-THPC.

Results

FaDu cells incubated with Photosan III and mTHPC in the absence of light showed a decrease of cell viability correlated to photosensitizer concentration and incubation time. Cells incubated with 0.5 µg/ml Photosan III or 0.5 µg/ml mTHPC for 24 h did not show a significant difference in viability compared to untreated cells. The LD_{50} (at 24 h incubation time) of mTHPC was at a concentration of 2.5 µg/ml while it was 5 µg/ml with Photosan III. After incubation with 10 µg/ml Photosan III or 5 µg/ml mTHPC for 72 h, no viable cells could be observed.

The effects of illuminating the tumor cells after the addition of the drug are shown in figure 1. It is apparent that irradiation with 8 J/cm² of 630 nm light in the Photosan III group caused a 50% tumor cell death, while irradiation with 2 J/cm² of 650 nm light in the mTHPC group was sufficient to reach a 70% tumor cell destruction.

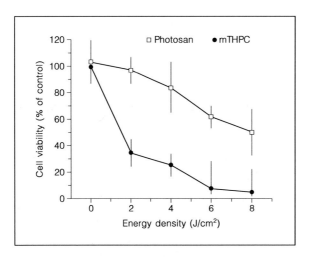

Fig. 1. The effect of Photosan III and mTHPC on hypopharyngeal carcinoma cells after irradiation. The points show the mean viability ± SEM of three cell culture plates. Incubation time = 24 h; wavelength: Photosan 630 nm, mTHPC 650 nm; sensitizer concentration: 0.5 µg/ml.

Our results indicate that the tumoricidal effect depends on photosensitizer dose and light dose.

Discussion

The goal of PDT is selective tumor eradication whilst sparing adjacent normal tissue. A sensitizer with preferential uptake by tumor tissue is administered and activated by a nonthermal dose of laser light of a specific wavelength leading to free radical formation and destruction of the target tissue. To overcome the shortcomings of HPD, new sensitizers have been developed with improved properties in this respect [8]. Among the chlorins, mTHPC has shown good tumor destruction and tissue selectivity in rodents, without apparent side effects and minimal skin sensitivity [9]. Furthermore, mTHPC strongly absorbs at 650 nm. This wavelength penetrates tissue better than that required for HPD activation.

Our initial aim was to test mTHPC in relation to Photosan III in a squamous cell carcinoma of the head and neck. This study was also designed to find appropriate substance concentrations for further animal studies in this kind of tumor. In our cell culture model, mTHPC seems to be at least 4 times more effective in photodynamic tumor destruction than Photosan III. Though the dark toxicity was twice as high as with Photosan III, we believe that deeper tissue penetration at 650 nm will compensate for this problem. Although mTHPC is considerably more potent on a molar basis than Photosan III, differences in therapeutic potency are not in themselves an over-riding consideration as they could be overcome merely by adjusting dosage. The limits on such adjustments are set mainly by toxicities for normal tissues, and thus the ruling consideration must be relative selectivity for tumors and normal tissues.

The mTHPC described here thus appears to be promising. Its therapeutic use in tumors of the head and neck will depend on further in vivo studies.

References

1 Berenbaum MC, Bonnett R, Scourides PA: In vivo biological activity of the components of haematoporphyrin derivative. Br J Cancer 1982;45:571.
2 Eichler J, Knopf J, Lenz H: Measurements on the depth of penetration of light (0, 35.1, 0 μm) in tissue. Rad Environ Biophys 1977;14:239.
3 Wan S, Parrish JA, Anderson RR, Madden M: Transmittance of nonionizing adiation in human tissue. Photochem Photobiol 1981;34:679.
4 Ben-Hur E, Rosenthal I: The phthalocyanines: A new class of mammalian cells photosensitizers with a potential for cancer phototherapy. Int J Radiat Biol 1985;47:145.
5 Chan WS, Svensen R, Phillips D, Hart IR: Cell uptake distribution and response to aluminium chlorosulfonated phthalocyanine, a potential antitumor photosensitizer. Br J Cancer 1986;53: 255.
6 Kessel D, Dutton CJ: Photodynamic effects: Porphyrin vs. chlorin. Photochem Photobiol 1984; 40:403.
7 Rangan SRS: A new human cell line (FaDu) from a hypopharyngeal carcinoma. Cancer 1972; 29:117–121.
8 Pandey RK, Bellnier DA, Smith KM, Dougherty TJ: Chlorin and porphyrin derivatives as potential photosensitizers in photodynamic therapy. Photochem Photobiol 1991;53:65.
9 Berenbaum MC: Comparison of hematoporphyrin derivatives and new photosensitizers; in: Photosensitizing Compounds: Their Chemistry, Biology and Clinical Use. Ciba Foundation Symp 146. Chichester, Wiley, 1989, p 33.

Dr. H. Heinritz, Department of Otorhinolaryngology, University of Erlangen, Waldstrasse 1, D–91054 Erlangen (Germany)

Rudert H, Werner JA (eds): Lasers in Otorhinolaryngology, and in Head and Neck Surgery.
Adv Otorhinolaryngol. Basel, Karger, 1995, vol 49, pp 48–52

....

Photodynamic Therapy of Superficial Skin Tumors following Local Application of Delta-Aminolaevulinic Acid[1]

H. Heinritz[a], *W. Benzel*[a], *R. Sroka*[b], *H. Iro*[a]

[a] Department of Otorhinolaryngology, University of Erlangen-Nürnberg, and
[b] GSF-Zentrales Laserlaboratorium, Neuherberg, Germany

Standard forms of photodynamic therapy (PDT) involve the administration of an exogenous photosensitizer [1]. If such a photosensitizer accumulates primarily within malignant tissues, later exposure to an adequate dose of photoactivating light may cause destruction of the malignant tissues without producing serious damage to the adjacent normal tissues.

The tissue photosensitizers that are in routine clinical use at the present are Photofrin II® and Photosan III®. These substances represent a semipurified complex mixture di-hematoporphyrinether and various porphyrin monomers and polymers. Both show a clinically useful degree of selective retention for many types of tumors compared to normal tissue (2:1 up to 4:1). But they also accumulate in liver, spleen, kidneys and skin [2]. Unfortunately, the accumulation in the skin leads to clinically significant photosensitization that persists for at least 3 weeks, and sometimes for several months. In this period, the patient is at risk of severe phototoxic reactions resembling that seen in patients with porphyria [3, 4]. This side effect is the major reason why PDT is not used much more widely. Consequently, there is a great need for new tissue photosensitizers that combine acceptably low toxicity and clinically useful tissue specificity without skin photosensitivity.

[1] Supported by the Johannes and Frieda Marohn Foundation, Erlangen.

Patients and Methods

Patients

Twelve patients with 12 superficial skin tumors in the head and neck area (10 basal cell carcinomas, two squamous cell carcinomas) have been treated with PDT in a clinical trial. To induce the synthesis of Pp IX we used a topical application of 20% ALA dissolved in propylenglycol and CAB-O-SIL (pH adjusted to 7.4 with $NaOH_3$). Following the application of the ointment on the tumor sites they were covered with a thin gauze and aluminum foil to prevent photochemical reactions.

Examinations

After complete ENT examination, each tumor was investigated by high-frequency ultrasonography. Ultrasound was used to define the lateral and axial extention of the lesions. Only tumors with an invasion depth less than 7 mm perpendicular to the skin were enroled in this clinical trial.

High-Frequency Ultrasonography

The ultrasonic investigations have been done in B-mode with the device 'DUB 20', taberna pro medicum, Lüneburg/Germany. This digital ultrasonic scanner allow elective investigation with 15 and 20 MHz. The 20-MHz scanner reaches a maximal axial resolution of 50 μm and a lateral resolution of 200 μm. The invasion depth varies between 7 and 15 mm and depends on the frequency and on the water content of the tissue investigated. The ultrasonic image is restored by attaching 256 different colors to the different echo amplitudes. The so-called 'wrong color coding' provides a much better discrimination of tissue structures than the conventional ultrasound working with 64 different grey values. The analysis of reflex patterns and echodensity enables tissue differentiation to be seen.

Fluorescence Measurement

In 6 of the 12 patients fluorescence measurement was done 24 h before PDT. Six to 8 h after ALA application, all tumors showed a maximum fluorescence intensity. According to these results, all patients were treated 6–8 h after ALA application. The measurement was performed with a self-constructed ratiofluorometric analyzer. For excitation, a HeNe-Laser (6 mW) was used. The fluorescence signal was detected at 665 nm with a combination of filters (RG 665) and a photomultiplier. Since a constant distance from the fluorometer and the tumor could not be maintained, the reflected laser light (632.8 nm) was also measured and related to the fluorescence signal. Conclusively, the 'ratiofluorometric signal' is largely independent of distance.

Treatment

At the maximum fluorescence intensity, the tumors have been irradiated with laser light of 630 nm (635 nm; see below) wavelength with 150 J/cm^2 and 100 mW/cm^2. An argon dye laser ('MDS 90', Aesculap-Meditec, Heroldsberg, Germany) was used as the light source.

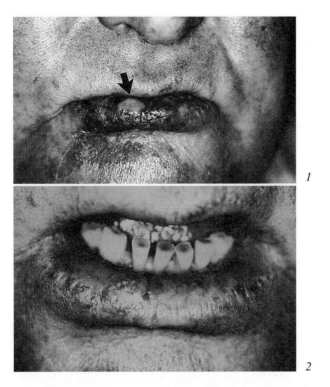

Fig. 1. Squamous cell carcinoma of the lower lip one day after PDT with ALA. A fibrinoid necosis (arrow) is delineating the former tumor margins.

Fig. 2. The same patient as in figure 1 4 weeks after PDT. The tumor has disappeared completely with a very good cosmetic result.

Results

Between 6 and 8 h after ALA application most tumors showed a fluorescence maximum which lasted up to 4 h and decreased slowly within the next 12 h. The lateral extensions of the tumors measured with fluorescence tend to be larger than with ultrasound. While the tumor margins appeared sharp on ultrasound they appeared blurred in fluorometry. In 2 of 6 cases, fluorescence was also detected beside the visible lesion. In these areas, evidence of subcutaneous tumor spread was confirmed by high-frequency sonography. The fluorescence of normal skin did not change significantly following ALA application.

Consequently, the treatment was performed 6–8 h after ALA application. The typical appearance of a squamous cell carcinoma one day after photodynamic therapy is shown in figure 1. Besides local skin irritation in the treatment area and minor pain during therapy, no side effects occurred. Four to 12 months after therapy, 10 of the 12 tumors including the 5 squamous cell carcinomas were histologically confirmed as complete, 2 were under partial remission and showed very good functional and esthetic results (fig. 2). The two basal cell carcinomas which initially showed a low fluorescence level persisted after photodynamic therapy. In 2 of the 10 cases of complete remission, the wavelength of the laser beam was adjusted to 635 nm because recently published reports gave evidence of increased photodynamic efficiency at this wavelength.

Interestingly, patients irradiated with 635 nm complained much more of pain at the tumor site than patients treated with 630 nm. The clinical results so far were not different in these two groups.

Fluorescence measurements before and after the treatment revealed a decrease in fluorescence immediately after irradiation. This may be due to the photobleaching effect. Within the next 2 h a slight increase of fluorescence was detected again, suggesting that some ALA had still been metabolized to Pp IX.

Discussion

As with any type of investigational treatment, the results must be compared with the current standard of therapy. The ideal treatment modality for head and neck malignancies combines tumor cell specificity with total tumor destruction. Unfortunately, no such modality currently exists.

The current standards of PDT as a selective tumor therapy regarding drug dosage, appropriate light delivery and optical dosimetry systems allow comparison of the results of different research groups. The high percentage of complete remission of superficial skin cancer following PDT with Photofrin II or Photosan III is combined with one major drawback: skin photosensitivity. Other side effects, i.e. nausea, vomiting, metallic taste, eye photosensitivity and liver toxicity, are rarely reported [5].

Protoporphyrin IX, an effective endogenous photosensitizer, obviously does not carry this side effect and currently leads to new enthusiasm in PDT [6, 7]. Our investigations reconfirm the absence of increased photosensitivity of normal skin following topical ALA application. We have also shown that endogenous protoporphyrin IX can be used for fluorescence diagnosis and for photodynamic treatment of superficial skin tumors at the same time. The ratiofluorometric system described above allows a quantitative fluorescence measurement of ALA-induced fluoresence in skin tumors. In combination with high-frequency ultrasound, it may be used to detect clinically invisible subcutaneous tumor spread and help define tumor margins. Since lesions with a low fluorescence level persisted after photodynamic therapy, fluorescence measurement may help select the skin tumors which are suitable for photodynamic therapy with Pp IX.

In photodynamic therapy of selected superficial basal cell and squamous cell carcinomas of the skin, topical ALA-induced Pp IX is very effective with high complete remission and excellent cosmetic results. The procedure has almost no side effects and can be done on an outpatient basis without analgesia or anesthesia. It is therefore especially suitable for multimorbid patients.

References

1   Doiron DR, Gomer CJ: Introduction; in Doiron DR, Gomer CJ (eds): Porphyrin Localization and Treatment of Tumors. New York, Liss, 1985, p xxiii.
2   Kessel D: Chemical and biochemical determinants of porphyrin localization; in Dorion CR, Gomer CJ (eds): Porphyrine Localisation and Treatment of Tumors. New York, Liss, 1984, pp 405–418.
3   Thomsen H, Schmidt H, Fisher A: Beta-carotene in erythropoietic protoporphyria: 5 years experience. Dermatologica 1979;159:82–86.
4   Mathews-Roth MM, Pathak MA, Fitzpatrick TB, et al: Beta-carotene therapy for erythropoietic protoporphyria and other photosensitivity diseases. Arch Dermatol 1977;113:1229–1232.
5   Dougherty TJ, Weishaupt KR, Boyle DG: Photodynamic therapy and early cancer; in De-Vita VJ, Hellman S, Rosenberg SA (eds): Principles and Practices of Oncology, ed 2. Philadelphia, Lippincott, 1985.
6   Kennedy JC, Pottier RH, Pross DC: Photodynamic therapy with endogenous protoporphyrin. IX. Basic principles and present clinical experience. J Photochem Photobiol 1990;6:143–148.
7   Kennedy JC, Pottier RH: Endogenous protoporphyrin IX: A clinically useful photosensitizer for photodynamic therapy. J Photochem Photobiol 1992;14:275–292.

Dr. H. Heinritz, Department of Otorhinolaryngology, University of Erlangen, Waldstrasse 1, D–91054 Erlangen (Germany)

Rudert H, Werner JA (eds): Lasers in Otorhinolaryngology, and in Head and Neck Surgery.
Adv Otorhinolaryngol. Basel, Karger, 1995, vol 49, pp 53–57

....

Photodynamic Therapy of Head and Neck Tumors

Jens Feyh

Klinik und Poliklinik für Hals-, Nasen-, Ohrenkranke, Klinikum Grosshadern,
Universität München, Deutschland

Photodynamic therapy (PDT) with a hematoporphyrin derivative (HPD) is increasingly being used in the clinic for the treatment of endoscopically or superficially remote malignomas [1, 2, 21]. Although this new treatment modality has been used in thousands of patients within the last 15 years, none of the studies that have been performed have shown a suitable place for photodynamic therapy in the clinical treatment of cancer in the future [3, 4]. According to the tissue penetration of light at the wavelength of 630 nm which is needed to excite HPD appropriately, every trial to treat tumors that are thicker than 0.7–1.0 cm will fail [5, 6]. Hence, a curative indication for photodynamic therapy is given for the treatment of T_1 and T_2 tumors only. In 1988, we started a clinical trial using photodynamic therapy as an exceptional therapy for T_{is}–T_2 cancers of the facial skin, oral cavity, oropharynx and larynx.

Besides this study, another study design has been conducted for the treatment of recurrent laryngeal papillomas in adults and children. HPV-associated papillomas are the most common benign laryngeal tumors in children and show a similar distribution in both sexes. Papilloma and condyloma are caused by the human papilloma virus (HPV) belonging to the family of papovaviruses [7]. Numerous studies have shown that there are at least 16 HPV subspecies apparent in man causing different deseases [8]. In children, papillomas of the larynx are histologically benign whereas in adults papillomatosis turns into cancer in 15% of the cases [9–11]. The conventional therapy is based on surgical removal of the papillomas by means of carbon dioxide laser systems. Because of the recurrent character of this disorder, the increasing number of surgical interventions leave scars in the mucous membranes of the vocal cords of the larynx. This results in increasing malfunction of the larynx.

All other treatment agents that have been added to surgery like steroids [8], aureomycin [12], idoxoridine [13], podophyllin [14], vaccine [15], and interferon [16] showed no significant effect to prolong the treatment interval of recurrent larynx papillomatosis.

Methodology

Fourty-eight patients meeting the inclusion criteria of the study design with a tumor in the head and neck area T_{is-2} were enrolled:

Face: 57 basal cell carcinomas and 7 squamaous cell carcinomas; oral cavity/oropharynx: 8 squamaous cell carcinomas; larynx: 11 squamaous cell carcinomas and 1 verrucous carcinoma.

Besides the tumor study, 24 patients with recurrent larynx papillomas were treated with PDT (14 adults, 10 children). Forty-eight hours prior to PDT, HPD (Photosan-3, Seelab, Germany) was administered intravenously. The laser light (630 nm) of an argon-pumped dye laser system (Meditec, MDS 90, Germany) was delivered via a 600-mm fiber-optic that was fixed in an optical device holding a spreading lens (Spindler & Hoyer, Germany) so that the laser beam could be spread to any size serving for a light homogeneity of ±3%. Light homogeneity was measured with photodiode (0.5 cm²) connected to a powermeter (Spectra Physics) in 10 different areas along the diameter of a laser beam spot (5 cm diameter). The laser light was applied 2 cm over each tumor edge if the anatomical site of the tumor allowed this procedure. All tumor sites received a total dose of 100 J/cm² at a power of 100 mW/cm².

From the time of injection of HPD, the patients remained in artificially illuminated rooms and were told to avoid sunlight for at least 4 weeks. Two months after PDT controlled biopsies in the former tumor area were taken from all tumor patients.

The integral laser illumination of the endolarynx for patients with laryngeal papillomas and larynx carcinomas was performed by means of a cylindrical laser light diffusor during laryngoscopy under general anesthesia. The light applicator system showed a laser homogeneity of ±5%. An argon dye laser system (Coherent, 630 nm) was used as a light source. All patients were treated with a light power density of 100 mW/cm², and a total energy amount of 100 J/cm². The duration of the laser light application was 16.6 min. After photodynamic therapy, the patients spent the first postoperative night in the intensive care unit.

Results

Macroscopically, all treated tumors responded completely to photodynamic therapy. Tumors of the skin showed strong extravasation directly after PDT. Twenty-four hours after laser treatment the treated tumor site was selectively covered by an eschar. Although the adjacent normal tissue was irradiated 2 cm over the tumor margin, only mild erythema was examined accompanied by a respectable amount of edema. The eschars disappeared continuously from day 13 after PDT onwards. The necrotic tumor sites epithelialized completely with excellent plastic results.

Tumors of the oropharynx responded to PDT in comparable tissue reactions due to the specific properties of the mucose membrane. Twenty-four hours after PDT, the tumor area was covered by a fibrin layer. The tumor surrounding and also irradiated normal tissue showed nearly no macroscopic alterations besides edema. From day 10 after PDT onwards, the necrotic tissue in the tumor area was rejected accompanied by substitution mucosal tissue. All treated sites epithelialized completely with excellent plastic and functional results. A similar effect were obtained in the treatment of laryngeal cancer. Mild edema occurred 24 h after PDT with no signs of dyspnea. Hoarseness of the patients lasted up to 6 weeks after PDT.

Over a longest follow-up of 5 years, 9 patients of this study showed histologically confirmed recurrence of disease. These patients were then treated by conventional surgery. This result is consistent with a complete response rate of 89.3%.

None of the patients with laryngeal papilloma showed laryngeal edema causing dyspnea following photodynamic treatment. Twenty-four hours after PDT, the papilloma tissue was livid and avital. Three to five days after PDT fibrinous layers could be observed in the former area of the papillomas. After 3–4 weeks, the endolarynx of all patients reepithelized without any signs of residual papillomas. In none of the cases treated could a synechia be observed. Over a longest follow-up of 34 months, 10 of 24 patients showed recurrence of disease within a relapse time of 4.4 months (7 adults, 3 children). All other patients still remain disease free.

Conclusion

The results of this study show, that photodynamic therapy can act as curative treatment modality for superficial cancer with excellent plastic and functional results. Additionally in most cases in the ENT-area no general or local anaesthesia is required.

Although thousands of patients have worldwide been treated with photodynamic therapy [2–4, 17, 18], the clinical value of this treatment modality still remains to be determined. This may be related to the fact that PDT is applied on tumor patients that have received every other conventional tumor therapy such as surgery, chemotherapy and radiation before PDT. Usually, the penetration of such tumors into the tissue is deeper than 1 cm, so that due to the tissue penetration of red light at the wavelength of 630 nm only palliation of these tumors can be expected [6]. Several reports on PDT show severe differences in the light energies and power densities of the applied red light within the studies so that a comparison of photodynamic effects between the treated patients of one study can hardly be obtained [19–21]. On the other hand, there are reports on the treatment of bronchial cancer by Hayata and co-workers [22, 23]. In this study, only early stage cancer of the bronchial tract has been treated with photodynamic therapy showing excellent results. Summarizing the experiences with photodynamic therapy by now, we must conclude that PDT is an adequate treatment for early-stage superficial cancer. Under these conditions and involving the patients in a prospectively randomized protocol using photodynamic vs. conventional therapy, it should be possible to prove the value of PDT in clinical practice.

Adult and juvenile recurrent larynx papillomas show macroscopic complete remissions following photodynamic therapy. No damage or scarring of the normal laryngeal tissue could be observed. The mechanism of the selective photosensitation of papilloma tissue still remains obscure. Although all patients showed papilloma disease with high recurrence rate in their medical history, only 42% showed a recurrence following one course of PDT. A similar distribution of the results was found in the group of adults and children. A selective impact of PDT on HPV-associated papillomas has been shown in animal experiments [24]. At present, little is known about the mode of action of PDT on papillomas. Probably, this tissue retains HPD to a higher degree opposed to the surrounding normal tissue because of its increased proliferation.

Based on these results PDT might be a hopeful tool for the treatment of recurrent laryngeal papillomas especially in children where often a tracheostomy has to be performed to prevent dyspnea. Further studies will show the value of photodynamic therapy to prolong the time interval for the treatment of recurrent laryngeal papillomas.

References

1   Berns MW, Wile AG: Hematoporphyrin phototherapy of cancer. Radiother Oncol 1986;7: 233–240.
2   Dahlman A, Wile AG, Burns RG, Mason GR, Johnson FM, Berns MW: Laser photoradiation therapy of cancer. Cancer Res 1983;43:430–434.
3   Carruth JAS: Photodynamic therapy: The state of the art. Lasers Med Surg 1986;6:404–407.
4   Gluckman JL: Photodynamic therapy for early squamous cell cancer of the upper aerodigestive tract. Aust NZ J Surg 1986;56:853–857.
5   Grossweiner LI: Optical dosimetry in photodynamic therapy. Lasers Med Surg 1986;6:462–466.
6   Svaasand LO: Optical dosimety for direct and interstitial photoradiation therapy of malignant tumors; in Doiron DR, Gomer TJ (eds): Porphyrin Localisation and Treatment of Tumors. New York, Liss, 1984.
7   Brandsma JL, Abramson AL: Association of papillomavirus with cancers of the head and neck. Arch Otolaryngol Head Neck Surg 1989;115:621–625.

8   Broyles EM: Treatment of laryngeal papilloma in children with estrogenic hormones. Bull, John Hopkins Hosp 1940;66:318–322.

9   Cohen SR, Geller KA, Seltzer S, Thompson JW: Papillomas of the larynx and tracheobronchial tree in children. Ann Otolar 1980;89:497–503.

10   Toso G: Epithelial papillomas. Laryngoscope 1971;78:1524–1531.

11   Yoder MG, Batsakis JG: Squamous cell carcinoma in solitary laryngeal papilloma Otolaryngol Head Neck Surg 1980;88:745–748.

12   Holinger PH, Johnson KC, Anison GC: Papilloma of the larynx: A review of 109 cases with a preliminary report of aureomycin therapy. Ann Otolar 1950;59:547–564.

13   Cook TA, Cohn AM, Brunschwig JP, Goepfert JS, Butel W, Rawls E: Laryngeal papilloma: Etiologic and therapeutic considerations. Ann Otolar Rhinol Lar 1973;82:649–655.

14   Dedo H, Jackler RK: Laryngeal papilloma: Results of treatment with the CO_2 laser and podophyllum. Ann Otol Rhinol Lar 1982;91:430–435.

15   Holinger PH, Schild JA, Mazurizi DG: Laryngeal Papilloma: Review of Etiology and Therapy. Laryngoscope 1968;78:1462–1474.

16   Schouten TJ, Weimar W, Bos JH, Bos CE, Cremers CWRJ, Schellekens H: Treatment of juvenile laryngeal papillomatosis with two types of interferon. Laryngoscope 1982;92:686–688.

17   Dougherty TJ, Lawrence G, Kaufman JE, Boyle D, Weishaupt DR, Goldfarb A: Photoradiation in the treatment of recurrent breast carcinoma. J Natl Cancer Inst 1979;62:231–237.

18   Dougherty TJ: Hematoporphyrin derivative for detection and treatment of cancer. J Surg Oncol 1980;15:209–210.

19   Harris DM, Hill JH, Werjgaveb JA: Porphyrin fluorescence and photosensitization in head and neck cancer. Arch Otolaryngol Head Neck Surg 1986;112:1194–1199.

20   Keller GS, Doiron DR, Fisher GU: Photodynamic therapy in otolaryngology: Head and neck surgery. Arch Otolaryngol 1985;111:758–761.

21   Sery TW, Shields JA, Augsburger JJ, Shah GG: Photodynamic therapy of human ocular cancer. Ophthalmic Surg 1987;18:413–418.

22   Hayata Y, Kato H, Konaka C, Ono J, Takizawa N: Hematoporphyrin derivative and laser photoradiation in the treatment of lung cancer. Chest 1982;81:269–277.

23   Hayata Y (ed): Laser photoradiation for Tumor Detection and Treatment. Tokyo, Igaku-Shoin, in press.

24   Abramson AL, Waner M, Brandsma J: The clinical treatment of laryngeal papillomas with hematoporphyrin therapy. Arch Otolaryngol Head Neck Surg 1988:114.

Dr. Jens Feyh, Klinik und Poliklinik für Hals-, Nasen-, Ohrenkranke, Klinikum Grosshadern, Universität München, Marchioninistrasse 15, D–81377 München (Germany)

Rudert H, Werner JA (eds): Lasers in Otorhinolaryngology, and in Head and Neck Surgery.
Adv Otorhinolaryngol. Basel, Karger, 1995, vol 49, pp 58–62

....

Photodynamic Therapy in Head and Neck Cancer

R. Kim Davis

Division of Otolaryngology, Head and Neck Surgery, and John A. Dixon Laser
Institute, University of Utah School of Medicine, Salt Lake City, Utah, USA

This paper provides a brief prospective of the interesting history of photodynamic therapy (PDT) in the treatment of head and neck cancer. The current
limited role of PDT will be discussed, and observations concerning its potential future use are given.

Phototherapy is a treatment modality wherein light-activated drugs are
used to both detect and eradicate cancer. Ideal photosensitizers must be solu-
ble and able to be readily and safely transported in blood, or rapidly absorbed
by topical application. These agents must have as high a degree as possible of
selective tumor localization, retention, and activation by light absorption. As
the range of light absorption in living tissues is mostly between 400 and
800 nm, the photoactive agents must have appropriate bands within this spectrum. Ideally, photosensitizers should be in the longer wavelength range to allow the deepest penetration of the activating light. When activated, the photosensitizer must produce fluorescence or tumor necrosis in vivo. Agents must
have low dark toxicity, or, in other words, low toxicity in the absence of light
activation. Agents must also have minimal phototoxicity.

Activating light sources must produce narrow bands of light in the appropriate light range at safe power density and total energy delivery.

Phototherapy with Porphyrin Compounds

The demonstration that porphyrin compounds have significant photodynamic effects in several different human tumor systems caused great initial sci-
entific interest, and stimulated expansive studies [1]. Porphyrin compounds

were found to cause photooxidative injury to the microvasculature sensitized by hematoporphyrin derivative bound to the vascular wall of endothelial cells in the perivascular stroma of tumors. Ultimately, Photofrin II (Photofrin Medical, Inc.), a purified porphyrin derivative, gained widest use in American clinical trials to include limited head and neck studies [2, 3].

As is often the case with the introduction of new therapeutic modalities, initial porphyrin clinical trials were conducted in patients with far-advanced cancer. Areas treated included dermal metastases from a variety of different tumor types, or large head and neck primary sites, or regional cancer recurrences which either could not be otherwise treated, or had failed more standard therapy with surgery, irradiation, and/or chemotherapy. In some cases impressive tumor response was seen, especially in dermal metastases of rather limited nature. Response rates from 0 to 40% were reported in these trials with advanced head and neck squamous cell cancer. Such clinical trials in advanced disease were ultimately shown to only offer minimal palliation, typically slowing tumor progression for only a few weeks. Occasionally, severe complications like carotid artery blowout were reported. Experience with superficial, limited volume head and neck cancer, on the other hand, showed more substantial response rates. Cancers treated included basal cell and squamous cell cancer of the skin, and carcinoma in situ, stage I, and less commonly stage II and III squamous cell carcinoma of the oral cavity, oropharynx, and larynx.

The actual limiting factor in photodynamic therapy for these lesions was the propensity to develop significant skin phototoxicity. As these early lesions are also easily treated by other less-morbid methods (CO_2 laser excision or irradiation), phototherapy never gained any significant clinical utility except in the treatment of multiple-lesion skin cancers like that seen in the basal cell nevus syndrome.

Attempts to selectively increase the concentration of photosensitizers in tumor cells while lessening phototoxicity have been investigated, but have failed to show significant benefit. An example of this is the study of liposomes as a carrier of photosensitizers in the attempt to enhance tumor concentrations of porphyrins [4]. Studies have also been directed at different hematoporphyrin compounds to include polyhematoporphyrin esters in the hope of decreasing phototoxicity and/or increasing treatment efficacy. These studies to date also have not shown significant benefit.

Topical application of hematoporphyrin derivative, dye hematoporphyrin ether, or polyhematoporphyrin esters has not been proven to be effective. The rationale for topical use is that more selective tumor localization could potentially occur without the systemic toxicity seen when these drugs are given intravenously. An interesting current development in porphyrin photosensitizers has come through the use of aminolevulinic acid (ALA). Administration of ALA leads to the endogenous synthesis of protoporphyrin IX, an effective photosensitizer, which accumulates somewhat selectively in tumors. Epithelial and gastrointestinal tract tumors have been treated in animal models and in selected patients with some tumor effect [5–7].

Animal experiments at the University of Utah have shown ALA to be efficacious when used topically. In contrast to DHE, when delivered intravenously, skin phototoxicity is significantly less with topical ALA administration. This approach to porphyrin phototherapy certainly holds promise and will be investigated extensively.

Intraoperative Phototherapy

One alternate approach to phototherapy with advanced cancer is to couple phototherapy with surgery. As photodynamic therapy with porphyrin compounds has clearly shown significant efficacy in limited disease, and as surgical resections in the head and neck in general require relatively narrow margins around the tumor, the concept of treating the tumor bed and a margin around the original tumor site with intraoperative phototherapy is being investigated.

Animal studies at the University of Utah School of Medicine have shown the potential benefit of intraoperative phototherapy. Narrow field resection of implanted C-1300 neuroblastomas in AJ-CR albino mice led to local recurrence rates of at least 80%. Intraoperative phototherapy with DHE reduced the local recurrence rate to approximately 20% [8]. Similarly, local recurrence following near total resection of radiation-induced fibrosarcomas in the same animal model leads to 100% recurrence rates. Treatment with either DHE intravenously or aminolevulinic acid topically as an intraoperative adjuvant therapy will decrease local recurrence rates dramatically (10–30%). As both of these agents have shown efficacy in treating limited squamous cell carcinomas of the head and neck, clinical investigation using DHE vs. ALA as intraoperative adjuvants are now being designed.

Intraoperative phototherapy could play a significant role in patients who have stage II or III oral cavity cancers for whom standard therapy would be open composite resection. Patients who refused standard therapy (open resection), but who are resectable transorally would be ideal candidates. Narrow-field CO_2 laser resection (excisional biopsy) could initially be performed. The tumor bed and surrounding tissues could then be treated with topical aminolevulinic acid. Photoirradiation of the area treated would then be accomplished to maximize destruction of potential residual microscopic disease.

After appropriate healing these patients could still undergo postoperative irradiation therapy. Studies investigating this approach will be accomplished.

Several Photosensitizers

Several different photosensitizers have been investigated outside of the porphyrin family in an attempt to improve photodynamic therapy. Acridine orange is activated at 488–514 nm and has been shown to be taken up intracellularly by tumors in high concentration. Maximum tumor uptake oocurs 30 min to 4 h after administration. This agent has potential use of an intraoperative photosensitizer due to the characteristics mentioned. Unfortunately, as maximum absorption is near 500 nm, the depth of penetration of photodynamic effect with this agent will not be great.

Another common substance which has been investigated in intraoperative phototherapy is methylene blue. Intravenous applications of methylene blue lead to rapid tumor localization in approximately 30 min. There is no uptake in skin or musculature. This agent is eliminated from the body of experimental animals in approximately 8 h. As methylene blue is activated at 664 nm, there is significantly greater depth of penetration of this agent. Studies at the University of Utah have shown significant tumor destruction in phototherapy with methylene blue which will lead to further investigation.

Further research almost certainly will need to include projects evaluating combination phototherapy. The combination of porphyrin compounds with intracellularly active agents like acridine orange or methylene blue should theoretically lead to greater tumor cell kill than any of these agents used alone.

Another avenue of promise in phototherapy is the combined use of chemotherapy and phototherapy. Some investigation has been done with adriamycin, known to have a chemotherapeutic effect in head and neck squamous cell cancer. Interestingly, this drug is photoactive, and preliminary studies suggest that photoactivation of adriamycin may lead to higher tumor cell kill rates than when this drug is used purely as a chemotherapeutic agent. The concept of coupling phototherapy with other chemotherapeutic agents also shows theoretical promise.

References

1 Dougherty TJ, Kaufmann JE, Goldfarg A, Weishaupt KR, Boyle D, Mittleman A: Photoradiation therapy for the treatment of malignant tumors. Cancer Res 1978;38:2628–2633.
2 Gluckman JL, Waner M, Shumrick K, Peerless S: Photodynamic therapy. Arch Otol Head
   Neck Surg 1986;112:949–952.
3 Harris DM, Hill JH, Workhaven JA, et al: Porphyrin fluorescence and photosensitization in
   head and neck cancer. Arch Otol Head Neck Surg 1986;112:1194–1199.
4 Davis RK, Straight RC, Keresati ZG: Comparison of photosensitizers in saline and liposomes
   for tumor photodynamic therapy and skin phototoxicity. Laryngoscope 1990;100:682–686.
5 Van Hillegersberg R, VandenBerg JW, Kort WJ, Terpstra OT, Wilson JH: Selective accumulation of endogenously produced porphyrins in a liver metastasis model in rats. Gastroenterology
   1992;103:647–651.
6 Kennedy JC, Pottier RH, Pross DC: Photodynamic therapy with endogenous protoporphyrin.
   I. Basic principals and present clinical experience. J Photochem Photobiol B 1990;6:143–148.
7 Grant WE, Hopper C, MacRobert AJ, Speight PM, Bown SG: Photodynamic therapy of oral
   cancer: Photosensitization with systemic aminolevulinic acid. Lancet 1993;342:147–148.
8 Davis RK, et al: Intraoperative phototherapy. Lasers Surg Med 1990;10:275–279.

R. Kim Davis, MD, Division of Otolaryngology, Head and Neck Surgery,
University of Utah School of Medicine, 50 North Medical Drive, Room 3C 120,
Salt Lake City, UT 84132 (USA)

Rudert H, Werner JA (eds): Lasers in Otorhinolaryngology, and in Head and Neck Surgery.
Adv Otorhinolaryngol. Basel, Karger, 1995, vol 49, pp 63–66

....

Experience with Surgical Laser Treatment of Tattoos and Use of the CO_2 Laser in Plastic Surgery

D. Katalinic

Privatklinik Dr. Katalinic, Nürnberg, Deutschland

Removal of Tattoos by the Argon Laser Technique

Treatment of tattoos constitutes but a relative indication for the present-day use of a surgical laser. This holds true for all laser units now on the market. Laser machines designed for the expressed purpose of treating tattoos are worthless from the practical and economical viewpoint.

Our technique of removing tattoos [1] by argon laser is a proven method and is applied routincly. The underlying principle of treatment is removal of the pigment particles from the tissue. We remove extensive tattoos with the argon laser in two treatment sessions 7 days apart. The procedure is carried out under local anesthesia. First, laser dermabrasion is performed with a continuous-wave beam at 4–6 W output. This is followed by treatment in two layers with a pulsed beam of 4–5 W power delivered in a sequence of 0.05–0.2 s. Aftertreatment over a 7-day period consists of administering fibrinolytic ointment Fibrolan®. One week later, the pigment particles are removed by excochleation under local anesthesia or using EMLA® ointment.

The results of this technique stand comparison with any rival method of removing tattoos. In our verdict it is better than any other, this, however, probably being a question of experience and technical skill.

CO_2 Laser as Surgical Knife

Of late, reports have been published and discussions held at various conventions, in which the CO_2 laser is compared with the scalpel and described as the ideal or better instrument for work in cosmetic surgery [2, 3]. This notion has drawn emphatic rebuttal from experienced laser specialists practising as cosmetic surgeons [4].

We first started testing the possibilities of using the CO_2 laser in cosmetic surgery about 17 years ago. Our experience as well as that of other clinics amounted to the CO_2 laser not offering any significant benefits over the scalpel as a cutting instrument. Thus convinced, no experienced and renowned cosmetic surgeon far and wide used the laser as a substitute for the scalpel then, nor have they done so to the present day. Because we shared this conviction by reason of our many years of experience with the most varied types of laser (argon, CO_2, dye, and Nd:YAG) in the area of cosmetic indications, we decided to re-examine our attitude toward the CO_2 laser as a surgical knife. During the past year we operated 33 patients either solely or partly with the CO_2 laser, using the most advanced super-pulsed CO_2 system delivering 40–60 W of output power. The surgery performed comprised blepharoplasty (12 patients), facelift (3), cosmetic breast surgery (8), abdominoplasty (4), and other cosmetic operations (6). In some instances, the operation was conducted on the first half with the scalpel and contralaterally with the CO_2 laser. Statistical interpretation has not been attempted, as the subjective findings do not lend themselves to statistical techniques and would only distort the true meaning.

Results and Discussion

Our past and present experience has been collated and is summarized enumerating the advantages and disadvantages of the use of the CO_2 laser in cosmetic surgery (table 1).

The distinct advantage of the laser, when used as a surgical knife, lies in its hemostatic effectiveness. In cosmetic surgery, this venerable benefit of the CO_2 laser, however, merits limited tribute. Modern-day methods assume scrupulous and complete arresting of bleeding at the operative site, which is readily attainable by conventional means. Therefore, this is an unnecessary and inappropriate place to apply the commendable hemostatic quality of the CO_2 laser. Trelles et al. [3] have no justification for his contention that retrobulbar hematoma and possible blindness resulting from inadequate hemostasis is not a liability in blepharoplasty when operating by laser but is a consequence of surgery with the scalpel (and without CO_2 laser). To begin with, it is known that retrobulbar hematoma usually occurs due to improper administration of local anesthesia (too deep and too coarse). Local anesthesia is still required when operating by laser. Secondly, this serious complication must be placed in correct relation to the millions of blepharoplasties performed by scalpel. The number of operations conducted with the laser is small and the figures given are not verifiable either, since only an extremely small group of physicians in the world make use of the CO_2 laser instead of the scalpel in cosmetic surgery.

As a cutting instrument, the CO_2 laser possesses insurmountable drawbacks for cosmetic surgery to the surface of the skin [5, 6]. These are directly associated with two parameters of the laser beam: its speed of light and its high temperature. Incision of the skin by laser is always uneven, exhibiting a jagged

Table 1. The CO_2 laser as a cutting instrument in cosmetic surgery

Advantages of laser knife	Disadvantages of laser knife
Noncontact technique*	More difficult handling*
Considerably less bleeding	Equipment sterilization difficulties*
Slight postoperative swelling*	Longer duration of operation
Minor postoperative pain	Imprecise line of incision
Good local sterility*	Scarring (cosmetic)*
	Risk of skin perforation
	Extended wound healing
	More assistance needed
	Generation of fumes
	Need for protective eyewear
	High cost

*Not capable of being clearly allocated and are subjected to discussion from various aspects.

line because every motion of the hand, be it ever so small, immediately results in three-dimensional deformation of the incision, since the laser beam's speed of light is not amenable to control by the human hand. By contrast, incisions made with the scalpel are smooth and extremely accomodating to the hand of the surgeon and human reaction. The CO_2 laser beam generates heat of a few thousand degrees Celsius and cuts a 2- to 3-mm wide path accompanied by thermal necrosis at local sites and at depths away from the incision. Under the electron microscope these necroses are strikingly demonstrable (University of Münster, Prof. Lehmann). Delayed wound healing and coarser postoperative scarring are direct consequences of making incisions with the CO_2 laser. These are the reasons compelling some cosmetic laser surgeons to do without the laser for incising the skin, preferring the scalpel instead.

The advantages and disadvantages of our finding (table 1) are marked by an asterisk to denote that the details thus indicated are not capable of being clearly allocated and are subject to discussion from various aspects. Use of the CO_2 laser in cosmetic surgery comes down to a morally questionable level: on the one hand are seen the capable, up-to-date cosmetic surgeons who work with this magic instrument, the laser, and on the other are the rest who don't and instead continue to operate with the humble scalpel. There are those who would seek their own gain at this low level while the medical truth is left unheard.

References

1   Katalinic D: Removal of tattoos by argon and CO_2 laser: Method and technique. Lasermedizin 1991;7:152–156.
2   Morrow DM: La blépharoplastie au laser CO_2 par rapport à la blépharoplastie au bistouri traditionnel. Rev Soc Fr Chir Esthét 1991;63:43–49.
3   Trelles MA, Sanchez J, Sala P, David L, Agerge P: Removal of lower eyelid fatbags using carbon dioxide laser. Lasermedizin 1991;7:146–150.
4   Mittelmann H, Apfelberg DB: Carbon dioxide laser blepharoplasty: Advantages and disadvantages. Ann Plast Surg 1990;24:1–6.
5   Katalinic D: Indications, limitations and success of laser systems in cosmetic surgery. Communication at the International Workshop on Advanced Technology in Plastic Surgery, Varese, June 11–13,1992.
6   Katalinic D: Laser CO_2 contre bistouri en chirurgie esthétique. La revue de chirurgie esthétique de langue française 1994;74:7–10.

Dr. Dimitrije Katalinic, Am Plärrer 35, D–90443 Nürnberg (Germany)

Rudert H, Werner JA (eds): Lasers in Otorhinolaryngology, and in Head and Neck Surgery.
Adv Otorhinolaryngol. Basel, Karger, 1995, vol 49, pp 67–69

....

Value of Laser Therapy for Vascular Anomalies

Freddy Schauss, Wolfgang Draf

Department of ENT Diseases, Head, Neck and Facial Plastic Surgery,
Städtisches Klinikum Fulda (Teaching Hospital of the University of Marburg)
(Head: Prof. *W. Draf*), Fulda, Germany

Many years ago, the laser was introduced for therapy of vascular lesions of the skin. This type of treatment is in the meantime well established for superficial vascular anomalies such as teleangiectasia, pyogenic granuloma, lentigines, spider angioma and cutaneous hemangioma. However, until now, the value of laser therapy for deeper vascular structures as subcutaneous hemangiomas is not well defined. This is partially because of the limited action of the laser in the depth. Even new laser systems have a limited penetration so their indication field covers more superficial vascular and pigmented lesions. With increasing experience one will learn which type of laser is adapted for which type of lesion [1, 2]. Another reason for this uncertainty is due to an addition of side effects, specially of the Neodym-YAG laser, actually the only one able to produce a somehow deeper thermic effect, but which works unspecifically and therefore leads to more or less visible scars on the skin surface [3, 4]. So the question regarding the best way of treatment of deep hemangiomas still remains.

Another problem which appears during the study of the literature is that there is no standardization in the classification of hemangiomas [4, 5]. Several classifications, clinical, anatomopathological and radiological, are used and make a comparison of different methods of treatment difficult. So as Mulliken [6], 1990, we think that a classification needs a clinical base. This is the reason why we prefer the terms 'cutaneous' and 'subcutaneous' hemangioma, giving an idea how deep the tumor extends whereas the classical terms 'capillary' and 'cavernous' are based on anatomopathological findings.

In this publication we want to concentrate on the treatment of hemangiomas. The following aspects should be considered when dealing with hemangiomas: (1) complete removal of the tumor so far as possible; (2) preservation of the function; (3) importance of good esthetic result.

Specially deep located lesions should be treated accurately to avoid recurrences. Because of scaring and changes in the connective tissue, a revision still presents more risks regarding the functional aspects, for example preservation of a nerval structure inside the tumor or of muscle mass as orbicularis oris. The best way to have functionally acceptable results is to avoid recurrences which means revisions. The esthetic result depends partially on functional integrity but also on the resulting visible scar. Based on these considerations, a therapeutic pattern was developed.

It is related to the depth of the tumor: superficial hemangiomas are treated with laser either alone in the case of cutaneous hemangiomas or in combination with surgery for mixed, it means both cutaneous and subcutaneous hemangiomas. Laser treatment is eventually applied in several sessions.

For subcutaneous hemangiomas extending into the depth, we see an indication for surgery with, as far as possible, a preoperative embolization [5]. In our opinion, transcutaneous laser therapy is not indicated here because of increased scaring of the skin. Intralesional laser irradiation is also not indicated because deep structures cannot be identified with certainty and could be injured. If a respectable blood loss is expected we like to use the cell saver which can wash the suckled blood and retransfuse it. With this procedure, even large tumors and those extending into the bone can be operated without major blood loss.

The extension of hemangiomas into the depth is actually best analyzed with a MRI. Besides, it facilitates the decision if a superselective angiography is indicated. During this procedure an embolization can be performed preoperatively or, in some cases, as arteriovenous hemangiomas, as definitive treatment. A high-resolution CT, in addition, is required for hemangiomas of the skull base or in the neighborhood of bone.

So the laser is one of the multiple therapeutic modalities to be included in a general concept. Most of time we use the Neodym-YAG-laser. A CO_2-laser is disposable for punctual lesions.

Between 1979 and 1993, we treated 99 patients with hemangioma. We began with laser therapy in 1988. Thirty patients were treated in 42 sessions. The hemangiomas were found 12 times on the lip, 5 times on the forehead, 4 times in the region of the eye lid, and three times each on the nose, tongue and cheek.

The technic used consists of application to several spots leaving bridges of intact tissue between the treated areas. To reduce the thermic damage, the skin is cooled with a wet, cold compress. Another possibility consists of laser through an ice block. Nevertheless, skin damage remains. We get the impression that the esthetic results depend on the localization of the hemangioma, probably subsequent to different tendencies of scar production. The mucosa shows generally good results even if an impressive swelling occurs during the immediate postoperative course. The esthetic results after laser on the skin of the lip and of the cheek are limited and less encouraging than on the forehead. On the helix, we could obtain a nearly inconspicuous scar.

References

1   Keller GS: Laser treatment of vascular skin lesions. Which laser: When, why, and how? Facial Plast Surg 6:1989;175–179.
2   Landthaler M, Braun-Falco O: Lasertherapie in der Dermatologie. Dtsch Ärtzebl 1991;31/32: 2638–2644.
3   Orenstein A, Nelson JS: Treatment of facial vascular lesions with a 100µ spot 577-nm pulsed continuous wave dye laser. Ann Plast Surg 1989;23:310–315.
4   Achauer BM, Vander Kam VM: Capillary hemangioma (Strawberry Mark) of infancy: comparison of argon and Nd:YAG laser treatment. Plast Reconstruct Surg 1989;84:60–69.
5   Apfelberg DB, Maser MR, White DN, Lash H, Lane B, Marks MP: Combination treatment for massive cavernous hemangioma of the face: YAG laser photocoagulation plus direct steroid injection followed by YAG laser resection with sapphire scalpel tips, aided by superselective embolization. Lasers Surg Med 1990;10:217–223.
6   Mulliken JB: Cutaneous vascular anomalies; in Mc Carthy JC (ed): Plastic Surgery, vol 5. Philadelphia, Saunders, 1990.

Dr. F. Schauss, Breslauer Straße 207, D–41366 Schwalmtal (Germany)

Rudert H, Werner JA (eds): Lasers in Otorhinolaryngology, and in Head and Neck Surgery.
Adv Otorhinolaryngol. Basel, Karger, 1995, vol 49, pp 70–74

....

Hemangioma: Differential Diagnosis and Necessary Early Laser Treatment

K. Schwager [a], *M. Waner* [b], *D. Höhmann* [a]

[a] Universitätsklinik und Poliklinik für Hals-, Nasen- und Ohrenkranke Würzburg
(Direktor: Prof. *J. Helms*), Germany;
[b] Department of Otolaryngology (Head: Prof. *J.Y. Suen*), Head and Neck Surgery,
University of Arkansas, Little Rock, Ark., USA

Vascular birthmarks are very common in children. Of every 3 newborn, 1 will have a vascular birthmark [1]. Most of them will fade or remain small and need no further treatment. One child in 100 will have a vascular birthmark that requires medical intervention. A major obstacle to our understanding and management of vascular birthmarks has been the nomenclature. The array of histologic and descriptive terms currently found in most texts lends little insight into the etiology, natural history and management of these conditions. An example of this confusion can be found in the generic use of the term hemangioma to describe an array of conditions that bare little or no relationship to one another apart from the fact that they are vascular in origin. These include strawberry hemangiomas and cavernous hemangiomas, lesions which typically show proliferation followed by involution. On the other hand, so-called capillary hemangiomas (port-wine stains), conditions that never show a hemangioma like proliferation or involution, or so-called 'cavernous hemangioma' which may refer to a venous malformation, are included in the term hemangioma as well. Mulligan and Glowatzki [2] recently proposed a biological classification of vascular lesions based on clinical behavior as well as cellular kinetics [2]. In accordance with this classification, two major types of lesions are recognized. These are hemangiomas and vascular malformations.

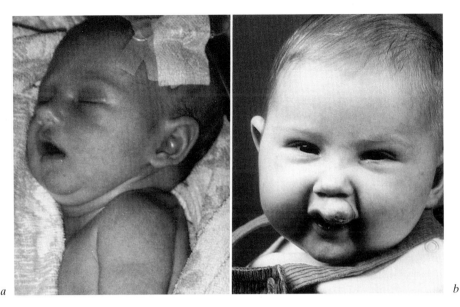

a   b

Fig. 1a. Starting proliferation of a hemangioma of the upper lip in an infant 1 week after birth. *b.* The same lesion at the age of 6 months.

The Natural History of Hemangiomas

Only 30% of hemangiomas are present at birth. The majority present during the first few weeks of life as an erythematous macule, a blanched macule or an area of localized telangiectasia often surrounded by a blanched hallow [3] (fig. 1a). The main characteristic of these lesions is proliferation during the first year of life [4] (fig. 1b). Two periods of rapid growth are frequently seen. One is during the neonatal period and in early infancy with a second period betwen 4 and 6 months of age. Especially the first proliferation period can show a very dramatic and rapid growth of the lesion. By the end of the first year of life, the proliferation stops and is replaced by involution. Histologically, this is seen as the proliferating plump endothelial cells become less active. They flatten progressively so that late in the process of involution, flat inactive endothelial cells predominate. Vascular channels become more and more obvious and large ectatic capillary-like vessels are seen [2]. In the end of the involution process, there are ectatic vessels surrounded by dense collagen and reticular fibers including islands of fatty tissue. Clinically, the hemangioma will become less tender to palpation during involution. A cutaneous hemangioma will change its colour from bright red to a darker, deep purple.

From the clinical aspect, 3 types of hemangiomas can be differentiated. Depending on its relationship to the skin, cutaneous, subcutaneous and transcutaneous or compound hemangiomas are recognized.

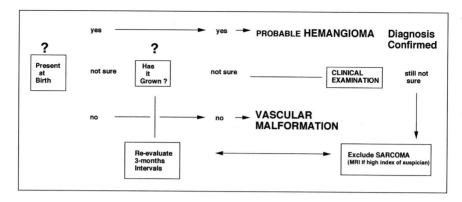

Fig. 2. Differential diagnosis of vascular lesions in early childhood.

The rate of involution is extremely variable. Bowers et al. [5] concluded that 50% of lesions will have involuted by 5 years of age and that a further 20% will have completed this process by age 7. In the remainder, complete involution may take a further 3–5 years. A very important issue concerns the degree of involution. Finn et al. [6] recognized 2 groups of hemangiomas, those involuted by 6 years of age and those that did not. In 80% of the lesions that had not regressed by this age, a significant cosmetic deformity resulted. Our own analysis of children with hemangiomas between 6 and 12 years of age revealed that cutaneous lesions were likely to leave epidermal atresia and telangiectasia. Subcutaneous lesions left a deformity due to residual fibrous fatty tissue and compound hemangiomas left a combination of epidermal atrophy, angiectasia and residual fibrous fatty tissue.

Differential Diagnosis of Other Vascular Lesions

A knowledge of the natural progression of hemangiomas is the paramount hint in differential diagnosis of other vascular lesions. Cutaneous lesions, like capillary ones such as nevus flammeus neonatorum or capillary-venous such as port-wine stains should be differentiated from cutaneous hemangiomas. The nevus flammeus neonatorum (salmon patch, angel's kiss, stork bite) is a transient, slightly red lesion. The most common site is the nape of the neck, followed by the upper eyelids, forehead, glabella, upper lip, and lower lumbar sacral area [7]. Most of these lesions fade within the first year of life, however the disappearance rate in the nape of the neck is much lower [8]. The port-wine stain is distributed in the head and neck region in relation to the branches of the trigeminal nerve. These lesions do not fade and have a tendency to become more ectatic and more obvious. Both lesions are true vascular malformations, i.e. they are present at birth, even though they may not be apparent, they never proliferate and therefore do not involute. Subcutaneous lesions are sometimes more difficult to assess and can be easily overlooked in a plump, well-nourished baby. Due to the possible fatal growth of hemangiomas, early diagnosis is necessary. Figure 2 shows a query for differential diagnosis of vascular birthmarks.

Treatment of Hemangiomas

The natural history of these lesions makes it necessary to intervene and treat these conditions as soon as they are diagnosed. For cutaneous hemangiomas yellow light laser treatment is recommended [9, 10]. Yellow light lasers have the advantage of good absorption by oxyhemoglobin and less absorption by melanin. As result, photocoagulation of the vessels can occur with less damage to the overlying skin [11, 12]. The flashlamp pumped dye and the copper vapor laser are feasible for these treatments, whereas the copper vapor laser seems to have advantages in the treatment of larger vessel disease, that can be found in hemangiomas [13]. In compound or transcutaneous hemangiomas only the cutaneous part can be treated by the yellow light laser.

Rapidly growing subcutaneous lesions can be problematic. Because they are too deep, they cannot be treated by yellow light lasers. The Neodynium:YAG laser can be used to treat this type of lesion. Especially in lip hemangiomas, the treatment can be done from the mucosal side in order to avoid cutaneous damage.

If there is a rapidly growing subcutaneous part or a subcutaneous lesion only, one should not hesitate in starting steroid therapy with prednisone. Signs of responsiveness should be seen within 7–10 days. Steroid therapy should always include a consulting pediatrician. In the period of involution, besides laser treatment, often reconstructive surgery has to be performed, in order to get a good cosmetic result.

Conclusion

It is necessary to differentiate between the various vascular birthmarks in children in order to provide adequate treatment in case of hemangioma or a vascular malformation. The rapidly growing hemangioma usually requires early treatment.

Typically hemangiomas start as small, unremarkable vascular lesions, but can grow rapidly. It is necessary to be aware of this sometimes fatal development. A small lesion during early proliferation can be easily treated with a yel-

low light laser. To avoid cosmetical deformity that would later require correc-
tive surgery, and to avoid serious complications, early yellow-light laser treatment is recommended.

References

1   Mulliken JB: Vascular malformations of the head and neck, in Mulliken JB, Young AE (ed):
    Hemangiomas and Vascular Malformations. Philadelphia, Saunders, 1988.
2   Mulliken JB, Glowacki J: Hemangiomas and vascular malformations in infants and children: A
    classification based on endothelial characteristics. Plast Reconstr Surg 1982;69:412–422.
3   Hidano A, Nakajima S: Earliest features of the strawberrymark in the newborn. Br J Dermatol
    1972;87:138.
4   Payne MM, Moyer F, Marcks KM, Trevaskis AE: The precursor to the hemangioma. Plast Re-
    constr Surg 1966;38:64–67.
5   Bowers RE, Graham EA, Tomlinson KM: The natural history of the srawberry nevus.
    Arch Dermatol 1960;2:667–680.
6   Finn MC, Glowacki J, Mulliken JB: Congenital vascular lesions: Clinical application of a new
    classification. J Pediatr Surg 1983;18:894.
7   Pratt AG: Birthmarks in infants. Arch Dermatol 1967;67:302.
8   Oster J, Nielson A. Nucha naevi and interscapular telangiectasis. Acta Paediatr Scand 1970;59:
    416.
9   Höhmann D, Waner M, Schwager K: Gelblichtlaserphotokoagulation vaskulärer Malforma-
    tionen im Kopf-Hals-Bereich. HNO 1993;41:173–178.
10 Waner M, Suen JY, Deinhart S: Treatment of hemangiomas in the head and neck. Laryngo-
    scope 1992;102:1123–1132.
11 Anderson RR, Parrish JA: Microvasculature can be selectively damaged by using dye-lasers: A
    basic theory and experimental evidence in human skin. Lasers Surg Med 1981;1:263–267.
12 Anderson RR, Jaenicke KF, Parish JA: Mechanisms of selective vascular changes caused by
    dye lasers. Lasers Surg Med 1983;3:211–215.
13 Waner M, Dinehart S: Lasers in facial plastic and reconstructive surgery; in Davis RK (ed): La-
    sers in Otolaryngology Head and Neck Surgery. New York, Saunders, 1990.

Dr. K. Schwager, Universitätsklinik und Poliklinik für Hals-, Nasen- und Ohrenkranke
Würzburg, D–97080 Würzburg (Germany)

Rudert H, Werner JA (eds): Lasers in Otorhinolaryngology, and in Head and Neck Surgery.
Adv Otorhinolaryngol. Basel, Karger, 1995, vol 49, pp 75–80

....

Nd:YAG Laser Therapy of Voluminous
Hemangiomas and Vascular Malformations

J.A. Werner [a], *B.M. Lippert* [a], *P. Hoffmann* [b], *H. Rudert* [a]

[a] Department of Otorhinolaryngology, Head and Neck Surgery
   (Chairman: Prof. *H. Rudert*), University of Kiel;
[b] Department of Otorhinolaryngology (Chairman: Prof. *K.-B. Hüttenbrink*),
   University of Dresden, Germany

Hemangiomas and vascular malformations can be treated successfully
with the laser [1]. Precise knowledge of the biophysical interaction between
the specific laser light wavelength and the respective vascular tumor is essential to profitably use the laser. There is no single type of laser that can achieve
equally good regression in all types of hemangiomas and vascular malformations. For the treatment of voluminous hemangiomas and vascular malformations, the Nd:YAG laser is particularly suited among all laser types presently
available for clinical use. It has a superior penetration depth when compared
to the hemoglobin-related absorption specificity of the yellow light lasers
which have a penetration depth of less than 0.5 cm. Successful treatment emi-
nently depends on the mode, the intensity and the duration of the Nd:YAG laser application. Uniform guidelines cannot be established since these parameters have to be modified for the respective type of hemangioma.

Cooling Techniques and Power Density

Nd:YAG laser light can cause extensive and uncontrolled thermal damage of the
skin and mucous membranes if applied without adjuvant cooling of the tissue. This damage may not be detectable during the initial application of the laser light. Exposed tissue
should therefore generally be cooled during Nd:YAG laser light application [2].

In cases where the hemangioma is located externally on the skin or in accessible regions of the lips and the oral cavity, cooling of the surface is easily done following the recommendations of Berlien et al. [3] by applying the laser light through an ice cube. The ice
should not contain too many air bubbles to avoid artificial scattering of the laser light. The
passage through the ice cube does not lower the Nd:YAG laser light power since water

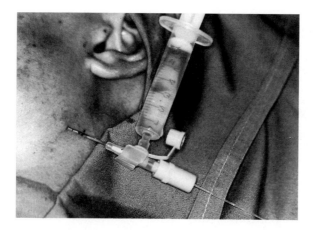

Fig. 1. Interstitial Nd:YAG laser light application in a vascular malformation of the left parotid gland. The laser light guide fiber is placed in the angioma through an i.v. cannula. The tip of the light fiber is irrigated with ice-cold Ringer's solution contained in the syringe. This is necessary during laser light application to prevent obstruction by blood clots.

only minimally absorbs light at a wavelength of 1,064 nm. Distant portions of the hemangioma may be reached by compressing the hemangioma with the ice cube [4]. This effect is particularly useful for the treatment of voluminous hemangiomas. The laser beam induces an increase in temperature in the hemangioma which in turn causes edema and beginning coagulation. The surface of the skin is only slightly harmed. Furthermore, vasculitis is caused with subsequent scaring of the vascular tumor.

Hemangiomas of the mucous membranes of the oral cavity, the oropharynx, the hypopharynx and the larynx require a different cooling technique. Cooling of the mucous membranes overlying the hemangioma is begun 10 min prior to laser light application. The patient has to be intubated and the head extended. The oral cavity and the pharynx are filled with ice-cold Ringer's solution which is exchanged several times. It remains inside during the use of the laser. Hemangiomas of the hypopharynx are exposed with a spreadable laryngoscope.

The laser light density used for the Nd:YAG laser therapy of voluminous hemangiomas and vascular malformations range from 500 W/cm^2 (equivalent to 2.5 W laser power and a spot size of 0.5 mm^2) to 3,000 W/cm^2 (15 W, spot size = 0.5 mm^2). The wide variation can be explained by the high variability of color, consistence and extend of the vascular malformation.

Ultrasound Guided Interstitial Nd:YAG Laser Therapy

Additional transmucous or transcutanous laser light application may be necessary in large hemangiomas if the external Nd:YAG laser irradiation can only reach a minor portion of the vascular tissue even when using the above-mentioned compression technique. A bare fiber is placed deep inside the hemangioma through a punction cannula or a punction catheter (fig. 1). The laser energy is applied directly to the tissue of the hemangioma

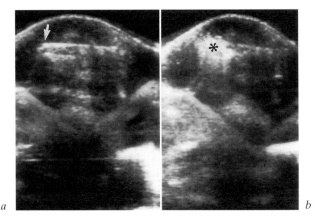

a   *b*

Fig. 2. B-sonographic control prior to (*a*) and after (*b*) interstitial Nd:YAG laser light treatment of a subcutaneous vascular malformation. The coagulated portion of the hemangioma can be identified by an increased echodensity (asterisk) at the tip of the laser light fiber (arrow).

while fiber and catheter are slowly withdrawn and the surrounding tissue is cooled by ice-cold Ringer's solution. The placement of the fiber is controlled manually and by ultrasound.

Interstitial Nd:YAG laser therapy guided by ultrasound allows treatment without major bleeding of even larger hemangiomas with a minimized risk, especially when compared to conventional surgical procedures. This method may also be used to treat hemangiomas located exclusively subcutaneously. The Nd:YAG laser light is therefore applied under B-sonographic control (fig. 2, 3) with a laser power of 4–8 W for up to 40 s (spot size = 0.5–0.6 mm). The laser light fiber is moved as soon as an increase in sonographic density is noted at the tip. Treatment should be finished when all areas of the hemangioma show an increase in sonographic density. A complete interstitial irradiation of the tumor is not possible if sensitive neighboring structures have to be protected against the Nd:YAG laser irradiation such as the orbita or the nasal skeleton in very young children. Close follow-up with ultrasound scanning is indicated in these cases for at least 2 weeks so that a renewed enlargement or revascularization starting from the noncoagulated areas of the hemangioma can be detected and treated early.

Extensive postoperative swelling often develops after Nd:YAG laser therapy of large hemangiomas and vascular malformations which can last up to 3 weeks depending on the size of the tumor. Perioperative antibiotics and postoperative steroids for 2–3 days reduce excessive swelling and inflammatory complications.

The postoperative involution period is followed-up for at least 3 months after Nd:YAG laser therapy of hemangiomas and vascular malformations. Repeated laser light application is indicated in cases with an increase in tumor size, insufficient regression or the above-mentioned revascularization following interstitial therapy.

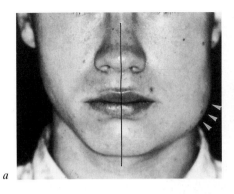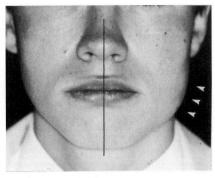

a

b

Fig. 3. Seventeen-year-old male patient with a vascular malformation of the left parotid gland prior to (*a*) and after (*b*) triple interstitial Nd:YAG laser therapy. Complete regression of the vascular malformation was not feasible because of a large vascular convolute located in the left vascular sheath. The patient was satisfied with the improved facial symmetry. —— = Axis of symmetry.

Results

Fifty-nine patients have been treated for 84 hemangiomas and vascular malformations at the Department of Otorhinolaryngology, Head and Neck Surgery, University of Kiel between 1987 and September 30, 1993. Twenty-three vascular anomalies had a minimum diameter of 3 cm in all directions. Complete clinical regression was accomplished in 14 of these 23 cases without any cosmetic or functional impairment. Six vascular malformations were reduced incompletely but satisfactorily for the patient. Two of the remaining 3 cases were treated by CO_2 laser surgery. Histology showed that Nd:YAG laser pretreatment had reduced the blood vessel component in both cases. The remaining angiomatous tumor was mainly formed by lymphatic vessels which did not regress because of the only minimal Nd:YAG laser light absorption of lymphatics.

Summarizing the results of Nd:YAG laser therapy of voluminous hemangiomas and vascular malformations one can conclude that this therapeutic concept achieves very good results if the recommended indications and techniques are observed. Therapeutic failure may be explained by a wrong irradiation technique or by a dominating lymphatic component of the vascular malformation.

Laser therapy is a highly successful form of treatment without major adverse effects for the patients and often with impressive cosmetic and functional results. The quality of these results justifies early laser treatment of hemangiomas and vascular malformations. This is especially true since hemangiomas have an unpredictable tendency to progress in 5–10% of the cases, partially with ulcerations. Depending on the location of the hemangioma life-threatening obstructions of luminous organs or compression of important structures may occur due to a fast increase in size.

Conclusions

Laser therapy of hemangiomas and vascular malformations can have excellent cosmetic and functional results as long as the type of laser is adequate for the type of vascular anomaly to be treated. Its high penetration depth makes the Nd:YAG laser especially suitable for the treatment of voluminous hemangiomas and vascular malformations.

The high penetration depth, on the other hand, can cause extensive thermal damage and subsequent scarring. Nd:YAG laser light should therefore only be applied with simultaneous cooling. Depending on the location this can be done with ice cubes or ice-cold Ringer's solution. The laser power density is set between 500 and 3,000 W/cm^2 relating to the intended tissue effect of the laser light. The aim is to irradiate until the vascular tissue turns pale. Carbonization should be avoided.

Ultrasound-guided interstitial Nd:YAG laser therapy allows treatment of large hemangiomas without major bleeding risk. The laser light fiber is inserted into the tumor with manual and sonographic control. Nd:YAG laser light is applied with a power of 4–8 W for up to 40 s. The position of the bare fiber is changed as soon as an increase in sonographic density is noted at the tip. The procedure should be finished as soon as all areas of the hemangioma appear to be sonographically dense.

Considering the good results, an early and consequent Nd:YAG laser light treatment of extensive hemangiomas and vascular malformations is indicated considering the good results. The often-quoted guideline of strict nontreatment for hemangiomas is not longer up to date since cosmetically and functionally disturbing scars may remain even after complete regression. In addition, progressive and regressive hemangiomas cannot be differentiated beforehand. Not least, one should save the patient and the parents from the sometimes immense psychical pressure.

Reference

1 Landthaler M, Hohenleutner U: Laser treatment of congenital vascular malformations. Int Angiol 1990;9:208–213.
2 Werner JA, Rudert H: Der Einsatz des Nd:YAG-Lasers in der Hals-, Nasen-, Ohrenheilkunde. HNO 1992;40:248–258.
3 Berlien HP, Waldschmidt J, Müller G: Laser treatment of cutan and deep vessel anomalies; in Waidelich W, Waidelich R (Hrsg): Laser 87 – Optoelectronics in Medicine. Berlin, Springer, 1987, pp 526–528.
4 Werner JA, Lippert BM, Godbersen GS, Rudert H: Die Hämangiombehandlung mit dem Neodym: Yttrium-Aluminium-Granat-Laser (Nd:YAG-Laser). Laryngo Rhino Otol 1992;71: 388–395.

Priv.-Doz. Dr. Jochen A. Werner, Department of Otorhinolaryngology,
Head and Neck Surgery, University of Kiel, Arnold-Heller-Strasse 14,
D–24105 Kiel (Germany)

Rudert H, Werner JA (eds): Lasers in Otorhinolaryngology, and in Head and Neck Surgery.
Adv Otorhinolaryngol. Basel, Karger, 1995, vol 49, pp 81–86

....

Therapy of Vascular Lesions in the Head and Neck Area by Means of Argon, Nd:YAG, CO₂ and Flashlamp-Pumped Pulsed Dye Lasers

Michael Landthaler[a], *Ulrich Hohenleutner*[a], *Talal Abd El Raheem*[b]

[a] Department of Dermatology, University of Regensburg, Germany;
[b] El-Menia University, El-Menia, Egypt

More than 30 years after the construction of the first laser by Maiman lasers are well established in dermatotherapy and the main indication for laser therapy are vascular skin lesions.

Biophysical Considerations

The argon laser is a continuous wave system emitting blue and green light (488 resp. 515 nm) that is absorbed in melanin and hemoglobin. This laser is therefore suitable for therapy of vascular and melanin pigmented skin lesions by rather unspecific epidermal and dermal coagulation. Applying short pulses (up to 0.3 s), the depth of coagulation is limited to about 1 mm. Vessel specificity of argon laser action can be increased by application of shorter pulses. Cooling the skin surface during laser irradiation reduces epidermal damage and, therefore, longer exposure times can be applied resulting in a coagulation depth of up to 3.6 mm [1–3].

The Nd:YAG laser emits in the near infrared range with a wavelength of 1,060 nm. Since melanin, hemoglobin, and water poorly absorb Nd:YAG-laser radiation, the energy penetrates deep into the skin resulting in deep coagulation up to a depth of 5–6 mm. Cooling the skin surface with water during Nd:YAG laser irradiation reduces epidermal damage and prevents vaporisation of tissue resulting in homogeneous coagulation. The depth of coagulation can be controlled by variation of laser power and time of exposure [4]. The Nd:YAG laser can also be used as a contact laser scalpel with artificial sapphire contact tips. Additionally, bare fibres can be introduced via puncture needles into thick hemangiomas for intratumoral coagulation.

The CO₂ laser is a continuous wave light source emitting infrared light at 10,600 nm. This radiation is strongly absorbed by tissue water, independent of the presence of chromophores like hemoglobin or melanin. The tissue damage created by the CO_2 laser is therefore nonspecific and its location and extent depend on the power density and the exposure time. The power density on the skin surface can be changed by simply moving the handpiece from and to the skin, i.e. focussing or defocussing the beam. A focussed small spot size and a high output power generate high power density resulting in vaporization and cutting of tissue.

Defocussing the laser beam gives a larger spot size with lower power density resulting in superficial tissue vaporization. Thermal damage to the adjacent tissue depends on the time of exposure and is limited to 0.3–0.6 mm. Cutting and vaporizing tissue by means of the CO_2 laser generates a tremendous amount of smoke which has to be removed by suction devices. This is mandatory since laser smoke might be a risk for the medical staff and the patients [5].

The flashlamp-pumped dye laser is a pulsed laser emitting yellow light at a wavelength of 585 nm, in pulses of 450 µs. Energy density can be varied between 6 and 10 J/cm^2. The use of this laser is based on the theory of selective photothermolysis [6], i.e. tissue targets absorbing the emitted wavelength may be selectively damaged if the pulse duration is shorter than the cooling time of the target. Therefore, this laser acts highly vessel specific in vascular lesions.

Clinical Applications

Port-Wine Stains (PWS)

Treatment of PWS is one of the most important indications for lasers in dermatology since there is no other comparably effective modality. The first laser, widely used for PWS, was the argon laser. Therefore, literature includes many papers concerning argon laser therapy of PWS. Good or excellent results of about 60% in adult patients are international standard [7–13] (fig. 1, 2). The results of argon laser therapy in 371 patients were significantly influenced by the patients' age, color and the local distribution of the lesion [9]. In about 48% of the patients under the age of 18 years good results could be obtained, in contrast to 70% in older patients. Only 30% of pink lesions responded to argon laser therapy in contrast to 70% of red and 75% of purple lesions. In about 70% of PWS on the head and trunk good or excellent results could be obtained compared to 27% on the legs. The size of the PWS had no significant effect on the outcome of the therapy but the best results were found in small lesions. Extensive PWS usually did not lighten homogeneously. For example, areas like the chin and the upper lip responded worse to laser therapy than the cheeks and the neck. Side effects of argon laser therapy were observed in 60 patients (16.2%): hypertrophic scars occurred in 4 patients (1.1%) and atrophic scars in 24 patients (6.5%). The latter usually adjusted to the surrounding skin in 6–12 months. Disturbances of pigmentation occurred in 32 patients (8.6%), in 26 hyper- and in 6 hypopigmentations. Based on these

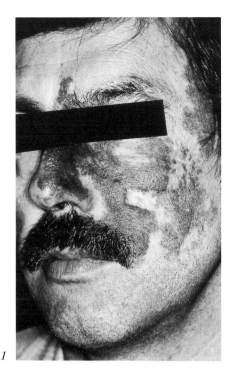
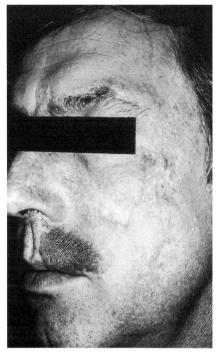

Fig. 1. Purple PWS in a 40-year-old male patient prior to argon laser therapy. Chronic radiodermatitis after X-ray therapy in childhood.

Fig. 2. Result of 12 argon laser treatments. Obvious lightening of the lesions; the bearded upper lip was not treated, clear difference between treated and untreated skin.

results we cannot recommend argon laser therapy for pink PWS and for patients younger than 18 years of age. Recently, however, the FPDL is of increasing importance in the therapy of PWS since this laser acts vessel specific and side effects are therefore rare. This laser is especially suitable for treatment of children and of pink and red PWS [14, 15]. In a study of our own, good or excellent results could be obtained with FPDL therapy of PWS in 60% of patients under 18 years of age. Side effects were infrequent and consisted mostly of transient hyperpigmentations [16]. Our results and the good results reported in the literature confirm that the flashlamp pulsed dye laser is the laser of choice for PWS treatment in young patients. But also in older patients with red PWS treatment results are superior compared to the argon laser.

In contrast, in purple PWS and PWS with nodular surface better results can be obtained by argon laser coagulation, in thicker lesions even by Nd:YAG laser coagulation or CO_2 laser vaporisation.

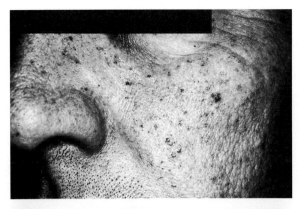

Fig. 3. Multiple venous lakes on cheeks and nose in a 60-year-old male patient.

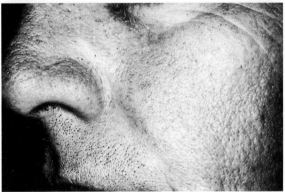

Fig. 4. Result of 2 argon laser treatments.

Telangiectasias

These lesions are an excellent indication for argon laser or FPDL treatment. We prefer the argon laser in patients with clearly discernible ectatic vessels, the FPDL if patients suffer from tiny vessels and a more diffuse redness of the cheeks. Results of both lasers are good or excellent in more than 80% of patients. Side effects of both lasers are hyperpigmentations.

Venous Lakes

These lesions are mostly located on the inferior lip and in some patients on the cheeks. They can be treated by argon laser coagulation with minimal side effects and excellent results. In thicker lesions up to three treatments are necessary, smaller lesions can easily be removed by one coagulation [17] (fig. 3, 4).

Adenoma Sebaceum

The small angiofibromas of Bourneville-Pringle disease can be removed with excellent results by argon laser coagulation or CO_2 laser vaporization.

Compared to dermabrasion, the advantages of laser therapy consist in the avoidance of general anesthesia and treatment on an outpatient basis. Treatment can be repeated easily and uninvolved skin can be spared out accurately [4, 10].

Hemangiomas

Since strawberry angiomas in children usually resolve spontaneously at the age of 6 years, indications for surgical or nonsurgical interventions were limited. Recent reports, however, clearly demonstrate that many patients may benefit from early laser treatment [18, 19]. Macular or flat elevated cutaneous hemangiomas often respond to FPDL therapy which is easy to perform and complications are rare [20, 21]. In some patients an obvious regression, in a few patients even a complete resolution, can be obtained. But one has to realize that the progression from cutaneous to deep hemangioma cannot be prevented in every patient [22]. Cutaneous or subcutaneous hemangiomas respond to Nd:YAG laser coagulation but these treatments can only be performed under general anesthesia. Small circumscribed hemangiomas can be coagulated by means of the argon laser or vaporised by the CO_2 laser. Laser therapy is indicated in hemangiomas of the face, especially of the eyelids, lips or nose.

Hemangiomas of the oral mucosa are excellent indications for Nd:YAG laser coagulation and complications are rare.

Conclusions

The introduction of lasers has dramatically improved the therapy of vascular lesions. Especially PWS can be treated but not all patients benefit from this treatment. Another important development is the early treatment of hemangiomas in newborns. In our experience there isn't one single laser that can be used for treatment of all kinds of vascular lesions. The FPDL is especially suitable for treatment of PWS in children and of pink PWS. However, the argon laser should be used for red and dark red PWS in adult patients, the Nd:YAG and CO_2 laser for purple PWS and PWS with a nodular surface. Therefore, the best treatment can be offered to patients if all different lasers are available and if the physicians are experienced with each of them.

References

1   Haina D, Landthaler M, Seipp W, Braun-Falco O, Waidelich W: Kühlung der Haut bei der Laserbehandlung von Gefässmälern; in Waidelich W, Kiefhaber P (eds): Laser/Optoelektronik in der Medizin. Berlin, Springer, 1986, pp 88–94.
2   Haina D, Landthaler M, Braun-Falco O, Waidelich W: Comparison of the maximum coagulation depth in human skin for different types of medical lasers. Lasers Surg Med 1987;7:355–362.

3   Hohenleutner U, Landthaler M: High power argon laser treatment of port-wine stains: Clinical and histological results. 1994; in press.
4   Landthaler M, Haina D, Brunner R, Waidelich W, Braun-Falco O: Neodym-YAG-laser therapy of vascular lesions. J Am Acad Dermatol 1986;14:107–117.
5   Landthaler M, Hohenleutner U: The CO_2-laser in dermatotherapy; in Steiner R, Kaufmann R, Landthaler M, Braun-Falco O (eds): Lasers in Dermatology. Berlin, Springer, 1991, pp 26–43.
6   Anderson RR, Parrish JA: Selective photothermolysis: Precise microsurgery by selective absorption of pulsed radiation. Science 1983;220:524–527.
7   Apfelberg DB, Flores JT, Maser MR, Lash H: Analysis of complications of argon laser treatment for port-wine hemangiomas with reference to striped technique. Lasers Surg Med 1983;2:357–371.
8   Cosman B: Experience in the argon laser therapy of port-wine stains. Plast Reconstr Surg 1980;65:119–129.
9   Landthaler M, Haina D, Seipp W, Brunner W, Seipp V, Hohenleutner U, Waidelich W, Braun-Falco O: Zur Behandlung von Naevi flammei mit dem Argon-Laser. Hautarzt 1987;38:652–659.
10 Landthaler M, Hohenleutner U, Donhauser G, Braun-Falco O: The argon laser in dermatotherapy; in Steiner R, Kaufmann R, Landthaler M, Braun-Falco O (eds): Lasers in Dermatology. Berlin, Springer, 1991, pp 44–59.
11 Noe JM, Barsky SH, Geer DE, Rosen S: Port-wine stains and the response to argon laser therapy: Successful treatment and the predictive role of colour, age and biopsy. J Plast Reconstr Surg 1980;65:130–136.
12 Ohmori S, Huang CK: Recent progress in the treatment of port wine staining by argon laser: some observations on the prognostic value of relative spectroreflectance (RSR) and the histological classification of the lesion. Br J Plast Surg 1981;34:249–257.
13 Seipp W, Haina D, Justen V, Waidelich W: Erfahrungen mit dem Argonlaser. Akt Dermatol 1981;7:106–114.
14 Garden JM, Polla LL, Tan OT: The treatment of port-wine stains by the pulsed dye laser. Arch Dermatol 1988;124:889–896.
15 Tan OT, Sherwood K, Gilchrest BA: Treatment of children port-wine stains using the flash-lamp-pulsed tunable dye laser. N Engl J Med 1989;320:416–421.
16 Hohenleutner U, Ahmed Abd El Raheem T, Bäumler W, Wlotzke U, Landthaler M: Nævi flammei im Kindes- und Jugendalter: Die Behandlung mit dem Blitzlampen-gepulsten Farbstofflaser. Hautarzt; in press.
17 Landthaler M, Haina D, Waidelich W, Braun-Falco O: Laser therapy of venous lake (Bean-Walsh) and telangiectases. J Plast Reconstr Surg 1984;73:78–81.
18 Apfelberg DB, Greene RA, Maser MR, Lash H, Rivers JL, Laub DR: Results of argon laser exposure of capillary hemangiomas of infancy: Preliminary report. J Plast Reconstr Surg 1981;67:188–193.
19 Hobby LW: Argon laser treatment of superficial vascular lesions in children. Lasers Surg Med 1986;6:16–19.
20 Garden JM, Bakus AD, Palles AS: Treatment of cutaneous hemangiomas by the flash lamp-pumped pulsed dye laser: prospective analysis. J Pediatr 1992;120:555–560.
21 Landthaler M, Hohenleutner U, Abd El Raheem T: Laser therapy of childhood hemangiomas. Br J Dermatol: in press.
22 Ashinoff R, Geronemus RG: Failure of the flash lamp-pumped pulsed dye laser to prevent progression to deep hemangioma. Pediatr Dermatol 1993;10:77–80.

Prof. Dr. Michael Landthaler, Department of Dermatology, University of Regensburg, D–93042 Regensburg (Germany)

Rudert H, Werner JA (eds): Lasers in Otorhinolaryngology, and in Head and Neck Surgery.
Adv Otorhinolaryngol. Basel, Karger, 1995, vol 49, pp 87–94

....

Suitability of Different Lasers for Operations Ranging from the Tympanic Membrane to the Base of the Stapes

R. Pfalz, R. Hibst, N. Bald[1]

University of Ulm, Department of Oto-Rhino-Laryngology, Ulm, Germany

Laser technology is in principle likely to enable more refined otological microsurgery on the ossicles. It is therefore surprising that no laser has become an indispensable instrument of surgery since the Nobel Prize was awarded in 1964. What are the reasons for this? It appears that no organ is as sensitive to bangs and heat as the ear. In addition, the organ of hearing is located very deep in the cranium, so that it is relatively inaccessible to experimentation.

The base of the stapes can be perforated with each of the four lasers, but the ossicles cannot be exposed. However, this can be carried out with the Er:YAG laser with almost no marginal damage. In his review article on the bone-cutting properties of very diverse infrared lasers published in 1988, Nuss et al. [1] already anticipated this. Hibst [2] analyzed in particular the Er:YAG laser in 1992. Monographs on the Er:YAG laser application and healing on the bone were published in 1992 by Hagemann et al. [3] and by Scholz Grothves-Spork [4]. Our experiments are based on these results and extend the figures with regard to thermal and acoustic limit values in operation on the bovine middle ear in vitro [5] and in anesthetized guinea pigs in vivo [6, 7].

First of all, I should like to recall some associations with regard to laser technology:

---

[1] Dedicated to my esteemed teacher Wolf Dieter Keidel.

(1) Coagulation entails thermal damage to hearing and balance. It is known that tenths of millimeters are significant under the base of the stapes in the organ of hearing and balance and that protein coagulates at about 56 °C. Thermal trauma comes to mind.

(2) Bubbles of steam are produced by the heat of the laser in the closed cochlea. They are likely to give rise to cavitation, exposure and trauma of the organ of Corti. In consequence of the formation and collapse of cavitation bubbles, pressure waves can arise which may lead to unpredictable damage in the closed network of pipes.

(3) Combustion of hydrocarbons and disturbance of wound healing by burnup metabolites are associated with carbonization. Furthermore, smoke obstructs the view and must be aspirated. However, one is also aware of the incalculability of the effect of the laser owing to variations in light absorption due to the blackening.

(4) In the context of resection of bone craters, one considers explosion, the thrust of ejected material, percussion trauma.

(5) With regard to energy, Watts or Joules, the layman thinks of enormous laser power, which cuts through armor plates. However, in reality, surgical lasers are too weak to cut bone more quickly than saws.

(6) The ideal of 'cutting without loss of tissue' can be implemented in bone only with the Er:YAG laser.

Although some surgeons have been successful [8–11], the argon laser can no longer be recommended [14–17]. On the one hand, its bone absorption is unpredictable and on the other hand it is subject to substantial transmission in the perilymph with injuries to the sacculus [12, 13]. Its thermal and acoustic characteristics would be acceptable for stapedotomy. Perforations of the ossicle would not heal because of the zone of coagulation, and they would become necrotic [18] (table 1).

In 1990, Lesinski [17] presented the long-term results of 153 stapedotomies carried out under local anesthesia with the super-pulsed CO_2 laser, beam diameter 0.5 mm, 3.6 W · 60 ms = 216 mJ. The stapedotomies were carried out to treat otosclerosis and the auditory results were improved. There were no reports of heat or carbonization, nor experience of bangs. Since the perforation should remain open in stapedotomies, healing of the wound was straightforward. With hot lasers, the channel obtained in the bone cannot be hollowed out to more than about 0.5–1 mm in depth because the carbonization blocks the channel and interrupts the supply of light. This is also not a problem at the thin base of the stapes. The energy is then transformed into heat instead of material removed.

The same applies to the Ho:YAG laser. Its emission (2.10 µm) is so far away from the absorption optimum of the bone that its absorption factor is only one hundredth of the Er:YAG laser. The transmission is 100 times greater (this is tolerable). Heating and carbonization occur [20]. The perforation channel is closed by drying out, blackening and silication below a depth of 0.5–1.0 mm.

The Er:YAG laser emits exactly the wavelength (2.94 μm) which is optimally absorbed by the water of the bone (13 %). The bone is removed mechanically. Very fine water droplets and vacuoles explode and disrupt the remaining particles without heating the very tiny microscopic particles from the crater. The light energy is consumed in transforming the vacuolar water from the liquid to the gaseous state. The perforation therefore has smooth walls with a margin of damage of only 20 μm. The hole punched out is round and empty at the bottom, so that a stable and reproducible effect and side effect is produced with the next bombardment. The energy is converted into removal of material, not into heat. The tissue remains almost cold. There is practically no coagulation and carbonization. Half of the energy is already absorbed after the laser has penetrated 1 μm into the perilymph. There is no transmission in the open labyrinth. A 0.2 mm beam of 50 mJ/0.25 ms requires 24 impulses to produce a channel depth of 1 mm. The channel produced is cylindrical and straight, so that an osteosynthesis wire can be led through it. As in a rocket propulsion the particles flying out of the crater cause an (acoustic) impulse in the opposite direction which is ≤ 1 ms, of a maximum of 133 dB(A) (at 200 mJ) and is transmitted to the chain. It sounds like a pistol shot: short and sharp (table 1).

In the center of the crater, the temperature is raised from 18 to 48 °C (spot diameter 1.7 mm) for 0.6 s after a 50-mJ impulse. One to two of these impulses are sufficient to perforate the base of the stapes. An impulse of 200 mJ also raises the temperature to 120 °C (spot diameter likewise 1.7 mm) for 0.6 s. The temperatures (table 1) were measured accurately on fresh bovine ossicles in vitro with a thermocamera (Probeye) to 1/8 mm with 20 images per second. With the Ho:YAG and Er:YAG laser, the heating takes place during the laser pulse. Since the pulse is so short, this therefore takes place during the duration of a single image taken with the thermocamera. The rise of heat up to the maximum requires one tenth of the time. The process of passive cooling requires nine tenths of the time. The rise time and the maximum temperature are important for the energy adjustment. The cooling time is important for the rate of laser repetition. Table 1 compares various lasers at energies which are just sufficient to perforate a normal base of the stapes. The heat at the center of the crater is shown in the column Tp_{max}. Only the Er:YAG laser remains below the coagulation point owing to its special mechanism of tissue removal. The bone material is expelled unchanged (cold) in microparticles of about 10 μm diameter from the crater. During the flight (towards the light), the particles are

Table 1. The Er:YAG laser works relatively cold on the ossicle and the base of the stapes

	Time of perforation ms	dB(A) peak	Tp_{max} °C	Increment/ decrement of temperature ms	Stapedotomy recommendation I/t/foc
Argon 1W/200 ms	160	91 (3.5 W/200 ms) chain	335	300/3,900	
CO₂ s.p. 15 W/50 ms [16, 17]	100 (1–3 pulses)	135 (15 W/50 ms) chain	420	100/10,000	172 mJ × n (SP · 3.6 W · 60 ms) human, focal distance 0.6 mm
Ho:YAG 200 mJ/0.200 ms [19] 250 mJ/0.250 ms [20, human]	0.5 (1–2 pulses)	138 (400 mJ/0.200 ms) chain	> 95	< 400/2,000	200 mJ × 2 in vitro focal distance 0.2 mm
Er:YAG 40 mJ/0.250 ms	0.2 (1–2 pulses)	133 (200 mJ/0.250 ms) stapes 153 (50 mJ/0.250 ms) ear drum/external, meatus	48	< 40/600	40 mJ × 2 in vitro focal distance 0.2 mm
ND:YAG, Q-sw. 25–31 mJ/100 ns [21, human]	6–12 bursts		athermic		
Excimer 7.5 mJ/20 ns [21, human]	0.160 (8 pulses)		athermic		

Left vertical column: laser parameters which just perforate the fresh base of the stapes (bovine, 0.2–0.6 mm). Column dB (A) peak: specifies in brackets the recommended duration of energy action and in dB (A) the acoustic peak and the site of laser application. Column 'increment/decrement': the temperature increment is followed by the highest temperature (Tp_{max}), and the subsequent cooling takes roughly ten times longer). The cooling time determines the selection of the impulse rate. Tp_{max} decides on the choice of laser and its energy parameters.

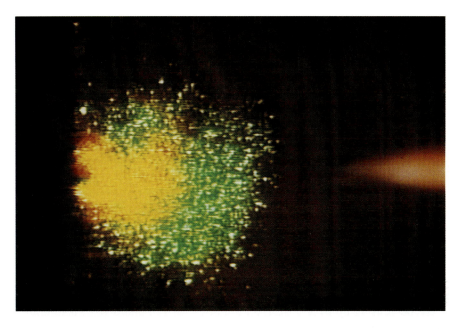

Fig. 1. High-speed photo of the removal process on the fresh femoral compact bone (bovine) during application of the Er:YAG laser impulse for 200 μs. Double exposure technique: 6 μs (yellow) and 11.5 μs (green) after the beginning of the impulse. Crater diameter (yellow) 100 μm. The bone particles removed cold fly towards the laser beam to the right (red). The vector, velocity and size of the particles can be estimated. The light emission derives from the particles (red-yellow-white luminescent particles) heated up by the (continuing) incident laser light during their flight. From Hibst [23].

warmed by the incident laser radiation. They can be identified on the basis of the thermal light emission (red) on the photo (as shown in fig. 1). A synopsis of the Er:YAG laser data on the dental enamel, dentin and bone has been presented in two publications [22, 23]. After osteotomy, this laser enables healing of the bone which is stable to loading stress [4], a characteristic which is not found after CO_2 laser osteotomies because of the ultrathin zones of silication, since the CO_2 light also conjugates onto hydroxyapatite.

Fresh bovine petrosal bones are suitable for in-vitro physical analysis of the laser bangs defined as peak × duration. This product also determines the acoustic risk for the hair cells. The acoustic risk can be appraised in accordance with the guidelines of the Federal German Army or the US Army, which were elaborated by Coles et al. [24] and Pfander and co-workers [25, 26]. We have reported on this evaluation [5]. In table 1, for comparison with other lasers the acoustic peaks are classified in dB(A) (for laser parameters which just perforate a normal base of the stapes). The application on the moist meatal mucosa in front of the limbus of the tympanic membrane is loudest. In the final analysis, determinations can be carried out only in vivo to establish the parameters (especially intensities) up to which the Er:YAG laser is without acoustic risk. We have compared audiograms before and after laser application in 44 anesthetized guinea pigs. These experiments were carried out on the one hand via the cochlear microphonics, and on the other hand via the BERA threshold [6, 7]. The impulse rate was increased with impulses of 50 mJ from 5, 10, to 25 and, finally, to 50, 100, 250 impulses. First (but temporary) reductions of the threshold by 38 dB (especially in the region of 2,000 Hz) only occurred after applying 500 × 50 mJ. There was complete recovery after 90 min. If the impulse rate is raised to 1,000 impulses of 100 mJ, there is little further increase in the depth of the trough, but this becomes broader in the direction of deeper and higher frequencies, and the recovery takes longer. We have obtained the same results with the BERA. After approval from the Ethics Commission, we have been using up to 500 Er:YAG impulses each of 50 mJ (0.25 ms impulse duration, rr 2/s, focus 0.3 mm) per ear in tympanoplasties. 500 × 50 mJ corresponds to the removal of 32 mg bone, i.e. roughly the weight of a malleus. We are on the very safe side with this dose, since guinea pigs are ten times more sensitive to impulses than humans [27]. This is also shown by the normal postoperative audiograms. The Er:YAG laser does not replace conventional methods in any situation, but only enhances them by a factor of 10 into the microscopic range, where the steady hand has natural limitations. We are thus breaking new ground and should avoid exaggerated enthusiasm.

Amongst the many applications which suggest themselves, tympanostomy under local anesthesia without tympanal tube has proved effective for evacuation of the mucoserotympanon. The patient hears a muted impulse of about 60 dB which is not unpleasant. After emptying the tympanum, the patient hears a normal pistol crack. The defect 0.3–0.5 mm in diameter closes after 3–8 days, depending on the diameter of the tympanostomy, and can be opened again in the doctor's office as required in order to blow the secretion via the Eustachian tube to the epipharynx in accordance with the technique of Rocco.

We have tested another application in 6 cases: the plug-socket connection between different ossicles (e.g. to raise the stapes by incus, anvil interposition or to anchor a wire prosthesis for malleo-stapediopexy).

In our experience, with these figures and cutting properties, the Er:YAG laser is proving itself as an almost athermal and acoustically controllable laser for surgery of the middle ear. Since this laser emits exactly the wavelength which the bone absorbs optimally, I cannot think of a more suitable laser. The

Er:YAG laser only passes glass fibers with a very muted signal. The zirconium-fluoride fibers (ZrF4) allow good conduction of Er:YAG light, but break easily, are expensive and possibly toxic. For this reason, the light must be applied via mirror arms. Since the Er:YAG light is invisible, a target beam is needed for aiming, which poses the difficulty to render the target congruent with the Er:YAG beam. This is a problem of physics which must be solved optically. I should therefore like to thank Zeiss (Oberkochen), especially Mr. Lasser and Mr. Reimer. I am also grateful to the Institute of Laser Technology in Ulm (Director: Prof. R. Steiner) for help in dealing with these problems of physics.

References

1 Nuss RC, Fabian RL, Sarkar R, Puliafito CA: Infrared laser bone ablation. Lasers Surg Med 1988;8:381–391.
2 Hibst R: Mechanical effects of erbium:YAG-laser bone ablation. Lasers Surg Med 1992;12:125–130.
3 Hagemann R, Walter JH, Zgoda F: Eigenschaften von biologischen Geweben; in Berlien H, Müller G (eds): Angewandte Lasermedizin. Berlin, Ecomed, 1992, pp II-3.1, II-3.4.
4 Scholz C, Grothves-Spork M: Die Bearbeitung von Knochen mit dem Laser; in Berlien H, Müller G (eds): Angewandte Lasermedizin. Berlin, Ecomed, 1992, pp II-3.1, II-3.4.
5 Pfalz R, Bald N, Hibst R: Eignung des Er:YAG-Lasers für die Mittelohrchirurgie. Arch OtorhinoLaryngol 1992:250–251.
6 Pfalz R, Nagel D, Bald N, Hibst R: Vergleich von BERA-Schwellen und cochleären Mikrofonpotentialen (CM) vor und nach Er:YAG-Laserung im Mittelohr narkotisierter Meerschweinchen. Vortrag 64. Jahresversamml Dtsch Ges HNO-Heilk, Kopf-Hals-Chir, Münster, 1993.
7 Pfalz R, Nagel D, Bald N, Stock K: Gehör (Cochleäre Mikrofonpotentiale) narkotisierter Meerschweinchen vor und nach Erbium:YAG-Laserung an Trommelfell und Mittelohr. Vortrag 9. Tag Dtsch Ges Lasermedizin, München, 1993.
8 McGee TM: Lasers in otology. Otolaryngol Clin North Am 1989;22:233–238.
9 McGee TM: Laser applications in ossicular surgery. Otolaryngol Clin North Am 1990;23:7–18.
10 Perkins RC: Laser stapedotomy for otosclerosis. Laryngoscope 1980;90:228–241.
11 DiBartolomeo JR, Ellis M: The argon laser in otology. Laryngoscope 1980;90:1786–1796.
12 Gantz B, Kishimoto S, Jenkins HA, Fisch U: Argon laser stapedotomy. Ann Otol 1982; 91: 25–26.
13 Silverstein H, Rosenberg S, Jones R: Small fenestra stapedotomies with and without KTP laser: A comparison. Laryngoscope 1989;99:485–488.
14 Lesinski SG, Palmer A: CO_2-laser for otosclerosis: Safe energy parameters – see comments. Laryngoscope 1989;99(suppl 46):9–12.
15 Lesinski SG, Stein JA: CO_2 laser stapedotomy (see comments). Laryngoscope 1989;99(suppl 46):20–24.
16 Lesinski SG, Palmer A: Lasers for otosclerosis: CO_2 vs. argon and KTP-532. Laryngoscope 1989;99:1–8.
17 Lesinski SG: Lasers for otosclerosis: Which one if any and why. Lasers Surg Med 1990; 10:448–457.
18 Pfalz R, Lindenberger M, Hibst R: Mechanische und thermische Nebenwirkungen des Argon-Lasers in der Mittelohrchirurgie (in vitro). Arch Otorhinolaryngol 1991;II:281.
19 Bald N, Göser C, Pfalz R, Hibst R: Akustische und thermische Wirkungen des Holmium:YAG-Lasers in der Mittelohrchirurgie (in vitro). Unpubl. 1992.

20 Hommerich ChP, Hessel St: Untersuchungen mit dem Holmium:YAG-Laser an Amboss und Steigbügel. Arch Otorhinolaryngol 1991;II:280–281.

21 Jovanovic S, Berghaus A, Schönfeld U, Scherer H: Bedeutung experimentell gewonnener Daten für den klinischen Einsatz verschiedener Laser in der Stapeschirurgie. Arch Otorhinolaryngol 1991 (suppl 2):278–280.

22 Hibst R: Lasereinsatz in der Zahnmedizin. Medtech 1991;18–23.

23 Hibst R: Mikrochirurgische Einsatzmöglichkeiten des Er:YAG- und Ho:YAG-Lasers am Knochen. In Vorbereitung.

24 Coles RRA, Garinther GR, Hodges DC, Rice CG: Hazardous exposure to impulse noise. J Acoust Soc Amer 1968;43:336–343.

25 Pfander F: Das Knalltrauma. Berlin, Springer, 1975.

26 Pfander F, Bongartz H, Brinkman H, Kietz H: Danger of auditory impairment from impulse noise: A comparative study of the CHABA damage-risk criteria and those of the Federal Republic of Germany. I Acoust Am 1980;67:628–633.

27 Rüedi L: Different types and degrees of acoustic trauma by experimental exposure of the human and animal ear to pure tone and noise. Ann Otol 1954;63:702.

Prof. Dr. med. R. Pfalz, Department of Oto-Rhino-Laryngology, University of Ulm, Prittwitzstrasse 43, D–89075 Ulm (Germany)

Rudert H, Werner JA (eds): Lasers in Otorhinolaryngology, and in Head and Neck Surgery.
Adv Otorhinolaryngol. Basel, Karger, 1995, vol 49, pp 95–100

····························

Application of the CO_2 Laser in Stapedotomy[1]

Sergije Jovanovic, Uwe Schönfeld

ENT Department, Klinikum Benjamin Franklin, Free University of Berlin, Germany

Stapedotomy is not only one of the most successful interventions in ear surgery but also one of the most dangerous for the inner ear. This explains the efforts made towards submitting the technique of stapes surgery to a critical analysis with the aim of minimizing its dangers. To reduce the risk of damaging middle and inner ear structures through manipulations with conventional instruments, the CO_2 laser beam is used for perforating the footplate and removing the suprastructures.

Since 1986, the application of the CO_2 laser in stapes surgery has been discussed in various experimental and clinical studies [1–11]. The clinical results illustrate the advantages of CO_2 laser stapedotomy. It is a noncontact technique that permits precise and controlled manipulation of middle ear structures. The CO_2 laser appears to be proving successful particulary for revisionary operations [4, 7–9]. One of the great advantages of the CO_2 laser is the high radiation absorption in the perilymph with the resultant low penetration depth of 0.01 mm. The argon and KTP laser beam, on the other hand, can spread out in the perilymph nearly unchecked but shows a high absorption in perfused tissue and pigmented cells. It can thus endanger inner ear structures.

[1] We wish to thank Laser-Medizin-Zentrum Berlin GmbH for technical support and Sharplan Lasers, Inc. for making available various new laser systems and high-precision micromanipulators. The work was supported by the Deutsche Forschungsgemeinschaft.

Materials and Methods

Criteria for the suitability of a laser in stapes surgery include its ablation rate at the footplate as well as the thermic and acoustic strain it exerts on the middle and inner ear.

These effects are the object of our investigations on isolated human stapes, in a simplified cochlea model and in animal experiments. The perforation diameters achievable at the footplate and the thermic effects are correlated with the laser-specific parameters of different laser systems and modes. We examined CO_2 lasers in the continuous-wave (cw) and superpulse modes. The laser parameters are selected to achieve an adequately large perforation of 0.5–0.6 mm.

Experimental Results

Owing to the high absorption of laser irradiation at 10.6 µm in bone tissue, the CO_2 laser yields highly reproducible perforations. An advantage of this laser is the possibility of achieving a sufficiently large perforation with one or several juxtapositioned applications.

The CO_2 laser is a thermically acting laser in the continuous-wave mode. Its thermic effect produces on the footplate adjacent to the perforation a glossy white crystallization zone, a dark brown to black carbonization zone and a golden brown thermic transition zone (fig. 1). A reduction of the beam diameter to about 180 µm markedly decreases the thermic side effects at the footplate. With this beam diameter, 4–6 juxtapositioned, partially overlapping applications are necessary to achieve an adequately large perforation of 0.5–0.6 mm (fig. 2).

The effect of the CO_2 superpulse system in the bone tissue is dependent on the intermediate power setting due to the given pulse-time behavior. The thermic effect of the CO_2 superpulse system is comparable to that of the CO_2 cw system with the same power density.

Apart from the suitability criterion ablation rate at the footplate and suprastructure, determination of the thermic and acoustic strain of the middle and inner ear during laser stapedotomy is of the utmost importance. We therefore investigated the local temperature rises in a caloric-physiologically approximated cochlea model under real perforation conditions of the stapes footplate. A high-speed videocamera operating at 1,000 images/s permitted the documentation of heat-transport mechanisms based on the thus-induced gas bubbles, which were already observed by Thoma et al. [11] in 1986. This yields convection-flow velocities of up to 0.1 m/s.

The temperature time course of local cochlear warming shows a rapid increase that reaches its maximal value at the end of the laser impulse. It is followed by a rapid convection-dependent cooling process with a subsequent

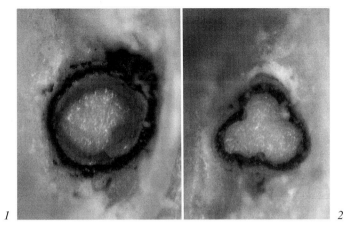

Fig. 1. CO_2 cw laser perforation of a stapes footplate (P = 18W/t = 0.05s/E = 6,000 W/cm^2; spot size = 0.56 mm).

Fig. 2. CO_2 superpulse laser perforation of a stapes footplate (P = 4W/t = 0.05 s/E = 16,000 W/cm^2; spot size = 0.18 mm).

slow phase. The local temperature elevations achieved with the CO_2 cw laser (P = 8 W; t = 0.05 s; E = 3,200 W/cm^2) are 15.2 °C (median) at a distance of 1 mm and 8.8 °C (median) at a distance of 2 mm behind the perforation.

With the superpulse mode, the temperature maxima are somewhat less marked at a comparable power density (13.1 °C in 1 mm and 4.6 °C in 2 mm).

The conditions on applying several laser shots in a 1-Hz rhythm show that there is a maximal temperature rise after each application. This does not, however, lead to a noteworthy summation of the temperature increments with a resultant increase in basal temperature.

Relating the maximal perilymph temperatures to the laser-beam diameter reveals a lower temperature elevation in the perilymph on application of a smaller beam diameter and the same power density. This is due to the lower energy required for a perforation when using a smaller laser-beam diameter. The CO_2 laser irradiation should therefore be applied with several shots with a small beam diameter, low power and short pulse times.

To examine the acoustic mechanisms of laser action in the cochlea, perforation of the footplate was likewise simulated in a simple model. A probe microphone linearized in frequency transfer function was connected to the 'round window'. Amplitudes and spectral distribution of recorded intra-cochlear pressure courses were compared.

Implosions of gas bubbles lead to impulse-like stimulations of pressure waves in the fluid. This results in a broad-band stimulation of the basilar-membrane. With the CO_2 cw laser, a noise signal is recognizable with increased amplitudes in the frequency range between 2 and 7 kHz. In the superpulse mode, on the other hand, the amplitudes are more pronounced in the low-frequency range, which largely reflects the stimulating pulse frequency of the laser.

Increasing power density involves a rise in the resultant pressures, which indicates a stronger basilar-membrane stimulation. Peak pressures of 22.4 Pa were measured for the CO_2 cw laser at a maximal power density of 7,200 W/cm^2. The influence of the pulse duration and the mode of application (perforating application or application in the open cochlea) on the measured pressures is negligible.

With the CO_2 superpulse laser, the measured sound pressures are more strongly dependent on the selected power density. In the superpulse mode, a higher mean power is archieved by an increase in the pulse frequency at a nearly constant pulse width and pulse peak power, that is, besides the higher power densities, the higher pulse frequencies lead to markedly higher pressure amplitudes. Peak pressures of 50.1 Pa were measured at a maximal mean power density of 4,200 W/cm^2. This renders the superpulse mode of the CO_2 laser less predictable in its effect and possibly more dangerous for the inner ear.

We have additionally investigated in vivo the effect of CO_2 laser irradiation on the inner ear using the laser parameters requisite for stapedotomy. The study was performed in female albino guinea pigs, and the site of laser application was the basal convolution of the cochlea. The aim was to examine the laser effect in connection with the perforation of the basal convolution and subsequent application in the open cochlea. Compound action potentials (CAP) were recorded. After application of the CO_2 cw laser three times at a power of 8 W (3,200 W/cm^2), a pulse duration of 50 ms and a repetition rate of 1 Hz (these parameters ensure an adequately large footplate perforation of 500–600 µm), the latencies of the CAP show no significant changes compared to the control group. There was likewise no threshold shift.

To test the application safety of this laser system, the power was increased to a maximal value of 15 W (6,000 W/cm^2) at the lowest possible pulse duration of 50 ms. These parameters did not lead to any CAP change. An increase of the pulse duration to 200 ms first caused changes in the CAP latencies that persisted up to the 14th day and were thus irreversible. An increase of the pulse duration to 500 ms ultimately led to hearing loss in all animals. These results show that the CO_2 cw laser is extremely safe for laser stapedotomy, since damage is only to be expected at much higher powers than those applied in clinical practice.

Table 1. Effective laser energy parameters for stapedotomy (Sharplan 1041 CO_2 laser)

Anatomic structure	Power W	Power density W/cm^2	Pulse duration	Operating mode	Number of pulses
Stapedius tendon	1	4,000	0.1	cw	3–5
Incudostapedial joint	5	20,000	0.05	cw	8–14
Posterior crus	5	20,000	0.05	cw	4–8
Footplate	2	8,000	0.1	cw	6–8
	4	16,000	0.05	cw	4–6

Focal distance: f = 250 mm; spot size: 0.18 mm (Acuspot 710).

Application of the CO_2 superpulse laser system in animals, on the other hand, already showed partially irreversible changes of the compound action in over 50 % of the animals within the effective laser range. Thus, application of the CO_2 laser in the superpulse mode with pulse peak powers of about 300 W for stapedotomy appears unpredictable and dangerous for the inner ear.

Clinical Experience

Table 1 shows the effective laser parameters determined for stapedotomy with the CO_2 cw laser. It appears advisable to us to select a small spot size (about 180 μm), low powers (1–5 W) and short pulse times of 0.05 s or 0.1 s in order to keep the requisite energy as low as possible.

The laser beam is conducted via a hinged reflector arm to the micromanipulator connected to the operating microscope and, from there, into the operating area. A favorable working distance proved to be 250 mm. The stapedius tendon is first vaporized with 3–5 single pulses at a low power of 1 W. The incudostapedial joint is then irradiated with the laser. With 8–14 single pulses of 5 W power, the stapes head is vaporized, thus releasing the joint. Then the posterior crus of the stapes is severed with 4–8 pulses at the same power. When severing the joint and the posterior crus with this relatively high laser power, care must be taken not to damage middle ear structures (footplate, facial nerve canal, etc.) lying in the beam direction. Reliable protection is provided by coverage with moist Marbagelan®. The anterior crus of the stapes is often not directly accessible to the laser beam; thus fracturing is done conventionally with the hook. It may be possible with the aid of a reflector to redirect the CO_2

laser beam in such a way as to permit vaporization of the anterior crus under visual control. The reflectors hitherto available were not yet optimal. Finally, the vaporization of the stapes footplate is performed with 4–6 applications of 4 W. The perforation diameters range between 0.2 and 0.3 mm for the single pulse, depending on the footplate thickness. A platinum Teflon piston 0.4 mm in diameter is then inserted in the perforation and fixed to the incus neck. Sixty-nine patients with otosclerosis have thus far been operated on with the CO_2 laser. In 4 cases, a revisionary operation was performed. None of the patients developed intra- or postoperative complications, nor did any of them sustain inner ear damage or display vestibular disturbance. No differences should be detected in the mean sensorineural hearing loss before and after CO_2 laser stapedotomy.

The great advantages of CO_2 laser stapedotomy are the noncontact, precise and controlled management of middle-ear structures, the facilitation of revisionary operations and the possible reduction of the incidence of inner-ear damage. Disavantageous are still the greater technical complexity and the presently unfavorable cost-performance ratio.

References

1   DiBartolomeo J: Argon and CO_2 lasers in otolaryngology: Which one, when, and why? Laryngoscope 1981;91(suppl 26):1–16.
2   Coker NJ, Ator GA, Jenkins HA, Neblett CR, Morris JR: Carbon dioxide laser stapedotomy: Thermal effects. Arch Otolaryngol 1985;111:601–605.
3   Jovanovic S, Prapavat V, Schönfeld U, Berghaus A, Beuthan J, Scherer H: Experimentelle Untersuchung zur Optimierung der Parameter verschiedener Lasersysteme zur Stapedotomie. Lasermedizin 1992;8:174–181.
4   Jovanovic S, Berghaus A, Scherer H, Schönfeld U: Klinische Erfahrungen mit dem CO_2-Laser in der Stapeschirurgie. Eur Arch Otorhinolaryngol 1992;(suppl II):249–250.
5   Jovanovic S, Anft D, Schönfeld U, Tausch-Treml R: Tierexperimentelle Untersuchungen zur Eignung verschiedener Lasersysteme für die Stapedotomie. Eur Arch Otorhinolaryngol 1993;(suppl II):38–39.
6   Jovanovic S, Schönfeld U, Fischer R, Scherer H: CO_2 laser in stapes surgery. Proc SPIE 1993, 1876:17–27.
7   Lesinski SG: Lasers for otosclerosis. Laryngoscope 1989;99(suppl 46):1–24.
8   Lesinski SG: Lasers for otosclerosis – which one if any and why. Lasers Surg Med 1990;10:448–457.
9   Lesinski SG, Stein JA: Lasers in revision stapes surgery. Oper Techn Otolaryngol Head Neck Surg 1992;3:21–31.
10 Lesinski SG, Newrock R: Carbon dioxide lasers for otosclerosis. Otolaryngol Clin North Am 1993;26:417–441.
11 Thoma J, Mrowinski D, Kastenbauer E: Experimental investigation on the suitability of the carbon dioxide laser for stapedotomy. Ann Otol Rhinol Laryngol 1986;95:126.

Dr. med. S. Jovanovic, Freie Universität Berlin, Klinikum Benjamin Franklin, HNO-Klinik, Hindenburgdamm 30, D–12200 Berlin (Germany)

Rudert H, Werner JA (eds): Lasers in Otorhinolaryngology, and in Head and Neck Surgery.
Adv Otorhinolaryngol. Basel, Karger, 1995, vol 49, pp 101–104

Results of Combined Low-Power Laser Therapy and Extracts of *Ginkgo biloba* in Cases of Sensorineural Hearing Loss and Tinnitus

P. Plath, J. Olivier

Department for ENT, Head and Neck Surgery of the Ruhr University Bochum, Prosper Hospital Recklinghausen, Germany

Since the end of the 1970s, several reports have suggested that low power laser therapy is effective on the improvement of wound healing: Later on, a combined therapy with a low power laser and extracts of *Ginkgo biloba* in the treatment of neurootologic diseases gained increasing consideration because of the need for conservative but intensive treatment of tinnitus as an extremely debilitating neurootological disease [1].

From September 1991 to June 1992, we accomplished a study designed as a blind trial of the efficacy of low-power laser therapy combined with extracts of *G. biloba* in the treatment of tinnitus.

Methods and Materials

Forty patients, 25 males and 15 females, with chronic tinnitus were admitted to the trial. All patients suffered from tinnitus for at least 6 months up to 5 years. Besides the tinnitus, all patients showed a sensorineural hearing loss, partially after sudden hearing drop. Before the trial, all patients had shown little or no response to a wide range of treatment including infusion therapy with hemorheologic drugs, iontophorese, acupuncture, and others.

Patients with dysfunction of the thyroid gland, cardiovascular diseases, or alterations of the upper vertebral column were not admitted to the study.

The patients were divided randomly into two groups:

Group A (laser group) underwent treatment with a low-power laser after injection of 50 mg *G. biloba* extract.

Group B (control group) received identical treatment with injections of *G. biloba* extract but only a sham laser irradiation.

Procedure and Posttreatment Analysis

Following the pattern of Witt [1], all patients received treatment, beginning with an injection of 50 mg *G. biloba* extract, followed by low-power laser therapy of the corresponding ear. The laser used was a combined helium neon (continuous wave, 632.5 nm, 12 mW output) and gallium arsenide laser (5 impulse regulated gallium arsenide infrared laser diodes, 904 nm, rated impulse power 30 W, frequency 100–2,800 Hz).

The distance between laser head and skin was 2 cm, the direction of the laser beam lead from 4 cm above the point of the corresponding mastoid to the lateral rim of the opposite orbita (i.e. close to the Schüller X-ray technique). The initial impulse frequency was 800 Hz with a daily increase of 100 Hz.

Treatment sessions for both groups were performed daily for altogether 8 days, and the laser irradiations (real or sham) lasted 8 min each. The control group also received an injection of 50 mg of *G. biloba* extract, the laser was positioned but switched so as not to transmit the laser beam.

Before starting the trial, in all subjects tone audiometry, tympanometry, and BERA where performed, as well as analysis for tinnitus in regard to its main frequency, loudness, and masking intensity of narrow band noise. In addition to audiometry, both groups received a scale for self-assessment, ranging from 0 (tinnitus as severe as before treatment) to 10 (complete relief). Audiometry and tinnitus matching were carried out after the 4th and 8th sessions, self-assessment after each session.

Results

According to the normal fluctuation of hearing test results, a reduction of tinnitus less than 10 dB was not accepted to be valued as a significant success. Also, a reduction between 10 and 20 dB is too small to be assumed as a significant difference. However, a reduction of 20 dB or more can surely be considered successful.

After treatment, the laser group showed a marked tinnitus reduction of more than 10 dB in 50 % compared with a reduction in only 5 % of the control group. A reduction of more than 20 dB was found in 6 subjects of the laser group, including 2 cases of complete relief. In the control group, only 1 subject showed a tinnitus reduction of 10 dB, higher reductions could not be achieved in the control group.

A relevant hearing improvement of 20 dB or more could be achieved in 1 subject of group A and in 3 subjects of group B. A change of more than 10 dB for the worse in hearing loss was not seen within either group.

Self-Assessment in Comparison with Audiometry

Comparing the self-assessment values with the audiometric results, a very good correlation could be found. In the laser group, 12 patients declared a reduction of tinnitus in the subjective scale compared with only 5 patients in the control group. A worsening of tinnitus was not stated by this method within both groups.

Control after One Year

One year after the trial, the 10 patients demonstrating subjective and audiometric improvement of tinnitus of more than 10 dB were asked to report their complaints matching them in the same manner by a self-assessment scale as within the study. All answered, but only 3 patients returned for audiometric control. In 2 of the 10 patients, the tinnitus reduction was assumed to be stable 1 year later and in 6 cases the reduction ceased with time. Two patients with only small primary effect reported that their tinnitus after finishing the trial returned to the extend it had before.

Discussion

The results of our investigation demonstrate that for the effectiveness of a low-power laser therapy in combination with injections of *G. biloba* extract, the zero hypothesis cannot be hold. In single cases, the tinnitus can be influenced positively by a significant reduction. This result is in good agreement with other reports mostly unpublished [1–5], which demonstrate the tinnitus unchanged in about 40 % of the treated cases, 45 % improvement of different degrees, and about 15 % relief of tinnitus at least for a longer time. In regard of the hearing function, the reported results are very different, but most authors did not see significant reduction of hearing loss.

In contrast to these reports is the result of a study from Walger et al. [6], who found no significant change in tinnitus and hearing loss, respectively. But this report must be refused for it was not performed under the direction and control of physicians but only by physicists. Therefore, the experimental order and the statistical analysis of the results are not in agreement with the rules of medical trials and statistics. The doses of *Ginkgo biloba* used were only homeopathic (D3), and the power of the soft laser was far beyond the effective range described by Warnke [7]. So these negative results, which also show reduction of tinnitus in single cases, cannot be accepted as an argument against the low-power laser therapy.

From the results of our experiment we assume that in single cases tinnitus reduction can be attained. Follow-up trials have to prove the influence of frequency and duration of the laser applications as well as of the *G. biloba* dosages. From the results of our study, we deduce that combined soft laser and *G. biloba* application can be helpful for some patients suffering from hard tinnitus.

References

1 Witt U: Low-Power-Laser und Ginkgo-Extrakte als Kombinationstherapie. Neue alternative Möglichkeiten bei Innenohrstörungen. Unpubl.
2 Goden H: Pers commun.
3 Kramp B, Bellin T: Pers commun.
4 Parthentadis-Stumpf M, Maurer J, Mann W: Softlasertherapie in Kombination mit Tebonin® i.v. bei Tinnitus. Laryngo Rhino Otol 1993;72:28–31.
5 Swoboda R, Schott A: Behandlung neurootologischer Erkrankungen mit Ginkgo biloba Hevert®, Hyperforat® und Low-Power-Laser-Therapie. Erfurt, 1992, unpubl.
6 Walger M, von Wedel H, Calero L, Hoenen S, Rutwalt D: Ergebnisse einer Studie zur Effektivität einer kombinierten Low-Power-Laser- und Ginkgo-Therapie auf den chronischen Tinnitus. Tinnitus-Forum 1993;III:10–11.
7 Warnke U: Der Dioden-Laser. Dtsch Ärztebl 1987;84:C-1824–1826.

Prof. Dr. med. Peter Plath, HNO-Klinik der Ruhr-Universität Bochum, Prosper-Hospital, Mühlenstraße 27, D–45659 Recklinghausen (Germany)

Rudert H, Werner JA (eds): Lasers in Otorhinolaryngology, and in Head and Neck Surgery.
Adv Otorhinolaryngol. Basel, Karger, 1995, vol 49, pp 105–108

....

Soft-Laser/Ginkgo Therapy in Chronic Tinnitus

A Placebo-Controlled Study

H.v. Wedel [a], *L. Calero* [b], *M. Walger* [a], *S. Hoenen* [a], *D. Rutwalt* [a]

ENT Departments of the
[a] University of Cologne, and
[b] University of Kiel, Germany

Soft-laser/Ginkgo therapy promised to be very effective in chronic tinnitus. This therapy consists of the combined application of soft-laser irradiation of the cochlea and the intravenous supply of Ginkgo extract 12 times in 4 weeks. Different studies reported beneficial results in 20–50 % of patients [Plath, 1992; Bellin, 1992; Swoboda, 1992; Zechner, 1993; personal communications]. But either the patient groups were very small or no placebo control was performed. We report the results of our study.

The effect of the soft laser is supposed to be an athermic stimulation of biochemical processes induced by light. Warnke [1] proved an increased ATP production in yeast fungus cultures irradiated with the soft laser. Whether these findings are transferable to human inner ear cells is purely speculative.

Materials and Methods

The laser we used (Medi HN 12-Combi, Fa. Felas) is a combined helium-neon/infrared diode laser. To reach the cochlea the laser has to penetrate 4–5 cm of tissue. Warnke [2] calculated that with this type of laser only 25 photons reach tissue at depths of 5 cm. In this regard, it does not seem very conclusive that there could be any therapeutic effect on human inner ear cells.

We performed the study on 155 patients with chronic tinnitus of more than 6 months' duration and with at least 1 or more unsuccessful treatments.

The patients were distributed into four groups, so that in case of therapeutic effect it is possible to differentiate between the laser and the Ginkgo effect and to see whether there is a synergism (table 1). Nineteen patients stopped the combination therapy, 6 of

Table 1. Study design

Group A	(n = 44)	laser active	Ginkgo i.v.
Group B	(n = 31)	laser active	NaCl i.v.
Group C	(n = 31)	laser inactive	Ginkgo i.v.
Group D	(n = 30)	laser inactive	NaCl i.v.

them because of tinnitus enhancement. These patients were excluded from the final evaluation of the results.

Before, after and 3 months after therapy we measured: audiogram, loudness of tinnitus, residual inhibition, tinnitus masking according to Feldmann, and evoked otoacoustic emissions.

On a visual analog scale (VAS) the patients had to indicate their subjective degree of loudness, annoyance and stress. The tinnitus questionnaire from Goebel/Hiller registered, in 52 questions, the patient's individual somatic and psychological handicap caused by tinnitus [3]. The subjective therapeutic effect was recorded by the questionnaire of Lenarz.

The treatment itself consists of twelve settings each 2–3 days. First 5 ml (>70 kg 10 ml) of a Ginkgo extract (Syxyl D3) are applied intravenously. A few minutes later the laser is activated in a position where the beam follows an imaginary line from the mastoid to the lateral border of the contralateral orbita. The pulse frequency of the diode laser is increased continuously from 1,200 to 1,800 Hz.

We also performed an experimental study to obtain the transmission values of the laser energy. Therefore, we placed a photo diode into the cochlea of 10 formalin-fixed human temporal bones without tissue. To avoid misleading effects of light the temporal bones and the photo diode were placed into a black box. The tension evoked in the diode, which correlates linearly with the laser power, is amplified and exposed on a voltmeter. Considering the lack of any tissue and blood supply, it is evident that the obtained values are higher than the real ones.

Results

Clinical Study

Tables 2 and 3 show the results of the direct impression of the patient, i. e. improvement yes or no, and of the psychometric questionnaire. It is very interesting that immediately after the end of the treatment 30 % more patients reported an improvement. This underlines the importance of a control months after treatment.

In tables 4 and 5, the results of tinnitus masking and audiograms are listed. An improvement of masking was defined as a decrease of 10 dB or

Table 2. Subjective impression	Improvement		Worsening	
	n	%	n	%
Laser/Gingko	3	7	3	7
Laser	2	6	4	13
Gingko	5	16	4	13
Placebo	2	7	5	17

Table 3. Psychometric questionnaire	Improvement		Worsening	
	n	%	n	%
Laser/Gingko	5	11	4	9
Laser	3	9	3	9
Ginkgo	3	10	0	0
Placebo	4	13	2	6

Table 4. Tinnitus masking	Improvement		Worsening	
	n	%	n	%
Laser/Gingko	5	11	4	9
Laser	3	9	3	9
Gingko	2	6	1	3
Placebo	3	10	2	6

Table 5. Audiogram	Improvement		Worsening	
	n	%	n	%
Laser/Gingko	2	4	0	0
Laser	1	3	1	3
Gingko	2	6	1	3
Placebo	2	6	2	6

more by masking with sinus tones or narrow band noise in the area of the tinnitus frequency. Improvement in audiograms corresponds to a decrease of 10 dB or more in at least 2 different frequencies. These changes have to be given special attention as they essentially concern patients with a pronounced hearing loss of more than 50 dB. All these results show only little differences between the groups and no tendency can be identified.

Laser Transmission Measurement

The Laser's helium-neon portion was completely absorbed. The values for the diode laser are at the lower limit of detectability. The registered values show a strong influence of pneumatisation on the mastoid. As reported below, the absorbing factors for skin, muscle and blood must be added to the results obtained and will lead to an additional decrease in power.

Conclusions

In all 4 groups there is improvement as well as worsening. No statistically significant difference can be seen.

The placebo effect has a great influence.

We cannot confirm the results of other studies. The fact that we used a Ginkgo preparation with a lower therapeutic dosage than other studies has been criticized, but this does not have an effect on the final results: the supposed 'repair mechanisms' are presumed to be activated by the laser *directly* on the flavo proteins *without* any interference by the Ginkgo. It should be kept in mind that the Ginkgo only provides a better oxygen supply. And even this could not be proven in experimental studies [4]. The patient's subjective replies seldom correlate with the audiologic findings. A standard evaluation protocol should be developed, which exactly defines the criteria of tinnitus improvement or worsening enabling better comparability between studies.

Certain criteria to identify possible responders could not be found.

The low power of the laser cannot achieve the postulated effects. Schnizer and Seichert [5] came to the same conclusion.

General application of this treatment for chronic tinnitus cannot be recommended, and it even seems dubious in individual cases.

References

1   Warnke U: Der Dioden-Laser. Dtsch Ärzteblatt 1987;84:24–26.
2   Warnke U: Wirkungsweise physikalischer Behandlungsmethoden (Infrarot-A-Laser, Ionen, Magnetfeld). Collegium veterinarium XXIII. Hannover, Schlüter, 1992, pp 150-154.
3   Goebel G, Hiller W: Psychische Beschwerden bei chronischem Tinnitus: Erprobung und Evaluation des Tinnitus-Fragebogens. Verhaltenstherapie 1992;2:13–22.
4   Lamm K, Arnold W: Sind durchblutungsfördernde Massnahmen mit Hämorheologica bei der Behandlung von Innenohrschwerhörigkeiten sinnvoll? Otorhinolaryngol Nova 1993;3:285–291.
5   Schnizer W, Seichert N: Lasertherapie: Eine kritische Betrachtung der sogenannten Soft- und Mid-Laserbehandlung. Med Welt 1988;39:1531–1538.

Prof. Dr. H. v. Wedel, ENT Department of the University of Cologne,
D–50924 Köln (Germany)

Rudert H, Werner JA (eds): Lasers in Otorhinolaryngology, and in Head and Neck Surgery.
Adv Otorhinolaryngol. Basel, Karger, 1995, vol 49, pp 109–113

....

Indications, Risks and Results of Laser Therapy for Recurrent Epistaxis

Godber Sönke Godbersen

Klinik für HNO-Heilkunde, Kopf- und Halschirurgie am Klinikum der
Christian-Albrechts-Universität, Kiel, Deutschland

Epistaxis is a common condition. 60% of the general population have one episode of nose bleed in their lifetime and 6% seek medical attention [1].

Recurrent minor epistaxis is not dangerous but inconvenient for the patient. The causes are often ectatic vessels or Osler's disease (hereditary hemorrhagic teleangiectasia). Conventionally, these patients are only treated during the actual episode using electrocoagulation or application of corresive substances. Laser light can induce histologic changes in blood vessels [2] and nowadays is a real therapeutic help in superficial vascular malformations [3, 4], gastrointestinal bleeding [5–8] and nosebleeding [9–11].

Materials and Methods

The Nd:YAG laser has been used at the Department of Otolaryngology, Head and Neck Surgery since 1989. Forty patients were treated for active or potential bleeding, 38 suffered from recurrent nosebleeds caused by ectatic vessels, 2 had Olser's disease. Patients with potential bleeding had ectatic arterial or precapillary vessels at the locus Kiesselbachii or similar changes in Osler's disease.

1% lidocaine containing 0.025% epinephrine was injected submucosally immediately before the operation. Besides the anesthetic effect this also improves the exposure of the ectatic vascular structures because the underlying tissue turns white. Superficial application of the anesthetic medication is not indicated since it causes vasodilatation and reddening of the mucous membrane which in turn unintentionally absorbs the laser light.

The laser light was applied for 0.3 s with a power of 10 W and a cable diameter of 0.6 mm. Actual bleeding was stopped by the application of several sorrounding spots (fig. 1). Laser light application to one point proved not to be good leading to scarification. An ectatic vessel which is not bleeding at the time of the procedure is coagulated by centripetal 'whipping' application of the laser light (fig. 2).

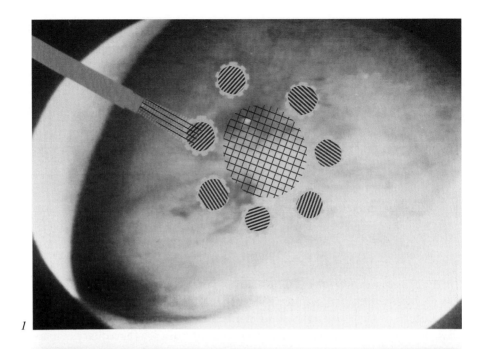

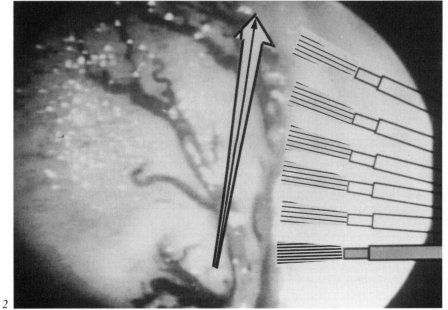

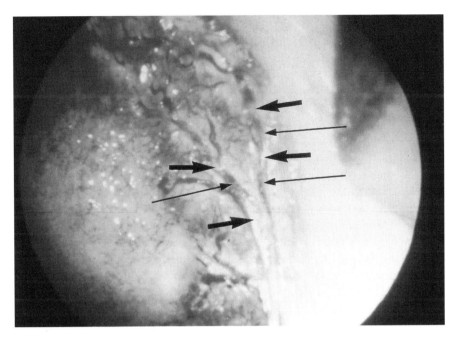

Fig. 3. Selected application of laser light to not acutely bleeding vessels results in ectasias (small and long arrows) between the coagulated portions (big and short arrows) of the artery and is therefore not recommendable.

Results

The results in cases of acute epistaxis occluding the vessels leading to the bleeding site by circled spots of the laser were not as good as following treatment in the sympom-free interval (fig. 1). The selected application of laser light to not acutely bleeding vessels results in ectasias between the coagulated portions of the artery (fig. 3). In more than 20 patients one procedure of laser light application was not enough so it had to be repeated 1 week later. Complications have not been seen. One of the patients with Osler's disease responded to the treatment. The other patient did not respond due to scarification following countless other procedures having been done before alio loco, like septodermoplasty, cauterization and nasal packings.

Fig. 1. Actual bleeding is stopped by the application of several surrounding spots. ⬬ = Laser light spots; ▨ = bleeding area.

Fig. 2. Laser light application to one point proved not to be good leading to scarification. An ectatic vessel which is not bleeding at the time of the procedure is coagulated by centripetal 'whipping' application of the laser light.

Discussion

In selected cases laser coagulation may help to prevent the initiation of a disastrous cascade of epistaxis therapy [12–14]. Today, different types of lasers are available which could generally be used for the sealing of blood vessels (Nd:YAG, 1,064 nm/argon laser, 480–514 nm /copper vapor laser, 588 nm). Most commonly utilized are the Nd:YAG [4] and the argon laser [9, 15]. An increase in temperature is caused by absorption of the laser light inducing coagulation with intravascular edema and thermal vasculitis subsequently causing obliteration. The respective biophysical properties of the Nd:YAG and the copper vapor laser are more suitable for the treatment of epistaxis than of the argon laser. Nd:YAG laser penetrates five times deeper into the tissue and four times deeper into the blood than the argon laser. The exposure time may be shorter since it has a higher laser power. Generally, the laser should be used in a noncontact mode to avoid coagulation of the surface of the mucous membrane and to minimize scarring and recurrences. Laser light application focussing on selected areas can only be recommended in Osler's disease [10] and in acute bleeding vessels. In these cases only the supplying vessels and not the bleeding site should be irradiated. Laser therapy in these cases with either the Nd-YAG or KTP lasers has been proven most efficacious before [11].

Risks can be ignored observing general precautions for the use of medical lasers. Special risks of the use of the laser for the treatment of epistaxis are perforation of the nasal septum and damage to the mucous membrane or the eye. To prevent septal perforation this procedure should only be done on one side since high temperatures may damage the mucous membrane. Injury of the eye can be avoided by the use of appropriate glasses (including the patient).

Conclusions

Laser coagulation proved to be a useful method to treat potentially bleeding lesions of the nose in patients with recurrent epistaxis. It is also beneficial in the management of active bleeding and in some cases of Osler's disease.

Laser therapy of epistaxis can be highly recommended in selected cases.

References

1   Shaw CB, Wax MK, Wetmore SJ: Epistaxis: A comparison of treatment, Otolaryngol Head Neck Surg 1993;109:60–65.
2   Solomon H, Goldman L, Henderson B, Richfield D, Franzen M: Histopathology of the laser treatment of port-wine lesions. Biopsy studies of treated areas observed up to three years after laser impacts, J Invest Dermatol 1968;50:141–146.

3   Enjolras O, Herbreteau D, Lemarchand F, Riche MC, Laurian C, Brette MD, Merland JJ: Hé-
    mangiomes et malformations vasculaires superficielles: Classification. J Mal Vasc 1992;17:2–19.
4   Werner JA, Rudert H: Einsatz des Nd:YAG-Lasers in der Hals-, Nasen-, Ohrenheilkunde.
    HNO 1992;40:248–258.
5   Fujimoto H: Endoscopic Nd-YAG laser therapy in upper gastrointestinal tract. Bull Tokyo
    Med Dent Univ 1988;35:59–61.
6   Cheng LH, Tsai WJ: Osler-Weber-Rendu disease: A six generation family. Kao Hsiung I Hsueh
    Ko Hsueh Tsa Chih 1992;8:495–502.
7   Buchi KN: Vascular malformations of the gastrointestinal tract. Surg Clin North Am 1992;72:
    559–570.
8   Selmeyer M, Cidlinsky K, Ell C, Hahn EG: Hämangiomatose der Leber bei Morbus Osler.
    Dtsch Med Wochenschr 1993;118:1015–1019.
9   Haye R, Austad J: Hereditary hemorrhagic teleangiectasia – argon laser. Rhinology 1991;29:
    5–9.
10 Davis RK: Lasers in otolaryngology: Head and neck surgery? Philadelphia, Saunders, 1990.
11 Siegel BS, Keane WM, Atkins JP, Rosen MR: Control of epistaxis in patients with hereditary
    hemorrhagic teleangiectasia. Otolaryngol Head Neck Surg 1991;105:675–679.
12 Deitmer T, Schürer G: Angiographische Embolisation als Alternative zur Unterbindung der
    Arteria maxillaris beim Nasenbluten. Laryngol Otol Rhinol 1993;72:379–382.
13 Hada Y, Hattori T, Seta H, Yanohara K, Kato A, Takahashi Y, Ono M, Ooi M, Nakagawa T:
    Embolization of internal maxillary artery for severe epistaxis-including an experience of ap-
    proach from superficial temporal artery. Nippon Igaku Hoshasen Gakkai Zasshi 1993;53:
    229–231.
14 Siniluoto TM, Leinonen AS, Kartunen AI, Karjalainen HK, Jokinen KE: Embolization for
    treatment of posterior epistaxis. An analysis of 31 cases. Arch Ololaryngol Head Neck Surg
    1993;119:837–841.
15 Illum P, Bjerring P: Hereditary hemorragic teleangiectasia treated by laser surgery. Rhinology
    1988;26:19–24.

Priv.-Doz. Dr. G.S. Godbersen, ltd. Oberarzt an der Klinik für HNO-Heilkunde,
Kopf- und Halschirurgie am Klinikum der Christian-Albrechts-Universität,
Arnold-Heller-Strasse 14, D–24105 Kiel (Germany)

Rudert H, Werner JA (eds): Lasers in Otorhinolaryngology, and in Head and Neck Surgery.
Adv Otorhinolaryngol. Basel, Karger, 1995, vol 49, pp 114–117

....

Carbon Dioxide Laser Delivery Systems in Functional Paranasal Sinus Surgery

Norbert Stasche [a], *Karl Hörmann* [b], *Matthias Christ* [a], *Horst Schmidt* [a, 1]

[a] ENT Department (Head: Dr. *N. Stasche*), Klinikum Kaiserslautern, and
[b] University ENT Department Mannheim (Head: Prof. *K. Hörmann*), Germany

The use of medical lasers is well established in ENT surgery, especially in laryngology. The carbon dioxide laser is the workhorse due to its favorable power and absorption characteristics, precise cutting and excellent control of tissue removal. The conventional use by handpiece or operation microscope in endonasal sinus surgery has various significant disadvantages, for example the necessity of a straight access to the target and the risk of accidental tissue damage. Flexible carbon dioxide laser beam delivery has become possible these days, although a lot of details need further investigation. The goal of this study was to evaluate different carbon dioxide laser delivery systems for paranasal sinus surgery, with special regard to their practicability and efficiency in everyday clinical use and their optical properties.

Material and Methods

In the ENT Department of the City Hospital, Kaiserslautern, 10 patients were submitted to laser surgery under a combination of local and general anesthesia. The systems employed were an operation microscope with a micromanipulator, a handpiece and three different waveguide systems. We tested Laprobe™, the ArthroLase™ and the Flexi-Lase™ system, in combination with a 20-watt-cw-carbon dioxide laser.

The Laprobe™ system consists of rigid, tubular waveguides, 300 and 450 mm in length and an outer diameter of 5 mm. It was originally developed for minimally invasive laparoscopic surgery. The components are an inner optical waveguide, a hollow light con-

[1] We thank Mr. P. Goedert, Department of Physics, University of Kaiserslautern, for support.

ductor made of special ceramics with metal coating and an outer metal protection sheath. Laser beam conduction is achieved by reflection on the inner ceramic surface.

The second rigid waveguide in this examination was the ArthroLase™ microguide system, originally developed for arthroscopic surgery. These hollow conducting probes are generally comparable to the Laprobe system described above. The working lengths are about 120 mm with a significantly smaller diameter.

The ArthroLase™ probes are available in a straight, a bent and a straight configuration with a 90° beam deflection.

The FlexiLase™ system is a flexible wave conductor, 120 cm in length, especially designed for the carbon dioxide laser. The construction principles are based on the development of flexible, inner mirrored hollow fibers, which allow a transmission of carbon dioxide laser light.

Before the waveguide systems came into clinical use, they were examined for transmission, beam diameter, divergency and power density. To measure the laser beam diameter, the 'knife-edge method' was employed, where a sharp edge is moved perpendicularly through the laser beam. Power transmission is measured depending on the edge's position.

Results

Operation Microscope

The operation microscope with micromanipulator provides an exceptional oversight of the operation site and precise focussing of the laser beam, which can easily be directed into the nasal cavity, but at the same time will only reach targets within the microscope's optical axis. Additionally, there is a considerable risk of accidentally burning structures of the nasal vestibule.

Handpiece

Lesions in the anterior part of the nasal cavity and extranasal pathology can be treated by means of the handpiece. It was clinically employed in the treatment of Osler's disease and rhinophyma.

FlexiLase

An energy transmission ranging from 50 to 60% can be achieved by this system. Consisting of a flexible fiber cable and a rigid handpiece, it was used in similar topographical situations.

Laprobe™

The transmission of this waveguide is about 75% and remains unchanged after single use. The permanent carbon dioxide gas rinse seems to offer sufficient protection for the probe from detritus and fluids from the operation site. The spot size can be varied between 0.8 mm next to the target and 2.9 mm at a distance of 30 mm. The probe tips allow a straight beam delivery or a 90° de

Table 1. Transmission values

Probe	Transmission, %
120 mm straight	77.0 ± 1.4
120 mm bent	79.7 ± 2.6
120 mm/90° deflection (new)	82.4 ± 1.8
120 mm/90° deflection (used)	24.6 ± 0.8

flection. In the measurement range from 0 to 30 mm away from the probe, a divergency of 1.38° ($\pm$ 0.15) was found. The minimum beam diameter was calculated 1.00 mm ($\pm$ 0.04). The power density was plotted against the distance. The maximum power density was 93 W/cm^2 ($\pm$ 30) measured directly at the beam discharge. Since the tip of the probe should not be in contact with the operation site, the practically achievable power density is estimated to be less.

ArthroLase™

All available ArthroLase™ probes were enrolled: a straight one, a bent one and a straight probe with a 90° beam deflection. Table 1 shows the transmission values.

All the transmission figures of the different probes in original condition were about 80%. Only the waveguide with a 90° deflection showed a clear decrease in transmission after being used twice.

The divergency was measured for the straight probe in comparison with the Laprobe series and is 2.33 ± 0.16 mm in the measurement range from 0 to 30 mm, yielding 0.66 ± 0.04 mm for the minimal beam diameter at the beam discharge.

The maximum power density per watt of the original output power at the beam discharge was 128 ± 46 W/cm^2, with corresponding reduction in practical use. The waveguide allowed employment in the paraendoscopic treatment of intranasal pathology.

Discussion

Operation microscope and handpiece are not considered to be ideal instruments for transnasal endoscopic laser surgery. There are imminent burn risks and a limited range of motion in dealing with hard-to-reach areas in paranasal sinus surgery. Both are of only limited use in this context.

The Laprobe™ system proved to be problematic for operating on such small cavities like the paranasal sinuses. The length of the probes and the outer diameter are developed to meet the necessities in abdominal surgery and gynecology, thus making a paraendoscopic endonasal approach almost impossible. The FlexiLase™ system did not withstand the clinical requirements. As the maximum transmission values do not exceed 50–65%, a relatively high input is necessary in order to obtain a power density that makes an efficient operating possible in a limited amount of time. In our case, this lack of performance led to inappropriate extension of operation time. Fenestration of the maxillary sinus could not be performed at all. In handling, the expectations of the new system were not fulfilled. Despite a flexible conduction cable, the connected handpiece is still rigid, impairing proper endonasal handling. Nevertheless, the cable can be moved much more freely, compared to the articulated arm, which means an important improvement, although this advantage might be more evident in free hand surgery than it is in endonasal procedures.

The ArthroLase™ delivery system offers a valuable improvement in having much smaller dimensions, thus making endonasal paraendoscopic working possible. Another advantage is the availability of a bent probe. It can easily be introduced into the nose or the trachea, even reaching areas out of direct visibility, especially when using the bent or the 90° deflection probe. This delivery system is the waveguide to be regarded as a true improvement to the microscope/micromanipulator combination.

We consider the ArthroLase microguide system to be most suitable for endonasal endoscopic carbon dioxide laser surgery, due to its handy dimensions, its satisfying power transmission, the avoidance of burn injuries and its ability to operate 'round the corner', even in topographically narrow areas.

Dr. N. Stasche, HNO-Klinik, Klinikum Kaiserslautern, Friedrich-Engels-Strasse 25, D–67653 Kaiserslautern (Germany)

Rudert H, Werner JA (eds): Lasers in Otorhinolaryngology, and in Head and Neck Surgery.
Adv Otorhinolaryngol. Basel, Karger, 1995, vol 49, pp 118–121

Reduction of Hyperplastic Turbinates with the CO$_2$ Laser

B.M. Lippert, J.A. Werner

Department of Otolaryngology, Head and Neck Surgery at the
University of Kiel, Germany

Nasal obstruction is a common disorder often caused by vasomotoric or allergic rhinitis. Its pathoanatomic substrates are enlarged inferior turbinates. Conservative therapeutic measures are often unsuccessful so that surgical treatment may be necessary [1]. Several different operative techniques have been described such as submucous turbinectomy [2], inferior turbinoplasy [3], conchotomy [4], total inferior turbinectomy [5], lateralisation of the turbinates [6], cryotherapy [7] and submucous diathermy [8]. Different types of laser have been used for reduction of turbinates in recent years with partly good results [6, 9–13]. Turbinate reduction with the CO$_2$ laser has been performed at the Department of Otolaryngology, Head and Neck Surgery at the University of Kiel since 1987.

Patients and Methods

Between April 1st, 1987 and January 31st, 1993, 76 patients have been treated for turbinate reduction with the CO$_2$ laser in a total of 172 operative procedures: 36 male, 40 female, average age 34.5 ± 7.3 years.

All patients were examined using both rigid and flexible endoscopes to estimate the extend of the hyperplasia of the turbinates and to exclude other pathologic changes. Preoperative rhinomanometry was performed to objectively measure the nasal obstruction and to ensure that it was caused by hyperplastic mucosa rather than by an enlarged turbinal bone.

The CO$_2$ laser light (mediLas Sharplan 1050, Sharplan Lasers, Germany, and OPMI-LAS CO$_2$50, Zeiss, Germany) was applied several times to the hyperplastic head of the turbinates without using vasoconstrictive substances. The laser was set at 1–4 W (depending on the micromanipulator), for a duration of 1 s. It was applied through the operating microscope (Zeiss OPMI-1, Zeiss) with a working distance of 400 mm. Until 1991 the 'Mikroslad 719' micromanipulator (focus diameter 0.64 mm, Sharplan Lasers, Germany), since 1992 the 'Acuspot 711' micromanipulator (focus diameter 0.25 mm, Sharplan Lasers, Germany) were used.

The operative procedure was mostly done in an outpatient setting and in local anesthesia in a combination of infiltration and surface anesthesia. Only in selected cases, e.g. in children or on request, was general anesthesia used.

All patients were examined postoperatively at weekly and later 3-monthly intervals. For 58 patients, a postoperative follow-up was made for 2 years. Endoscopy and rhinomanometry were performed. The patients were given a standardized questionnaire which was developed according to von Hacke and Hardcastle [14] and Warwick-Brown and Marks [15]. The following questions were asked:

(1) Was the operation successful for you?
(2) How long did the therapeutic effect last?
(3) Which symptoms were relieved by the operation?
(4) Did you observe any postoperative complications such as dry mucous membranes, nasal bleeding, unpleasant smell or incrustation?
(5) Would you again decide to have this operation?

To compare the long-term results of laser surgery with conventional therapeutic measures, we retrospectively examined 25 patients who were treated in 53 procedures by submucosal diathermy. Thirteen were male, 12 female with an average age of 29.8 ± 11.7 years. They all underwent endoscopy and rhinomanometry and answered the questionnaire.

Results

Nasal obstruction was already slightly improved a few days after CO_2 laser application. After 2 weeks a distinct effect could be shown. Postoperative wound care was necessary for less than 8–10 days in 90% of the cases.

Fifty patients (86.2%) who were treated by laser surgery were without complaints 6 months postoperatively. After 1 and 2 years, this applied for 48 (82.8%) and 46 (79.3%) patients, respectively. After submucosal diathermy only 17 (68%) patients were satisfied with the therapeutic outcome. After 1 and 2 years only 12 (48%) and 9 (36%) patients were without complaints. Postoperative complications were more common after submucosal diathermy than after CO_2 laser surgery. 50% of the patients treated with submucosal diathermy complained about extreme incrustation requiring extensive postoperative care. In 4 cases postoperative nasal bleeding was observed. The agreement to repeated treatment is different in 2 groups. 54 of 58 (93.1%) patients treated by laser surgery agreed to undergo repeated treatment. However, only 9 of 25 (48%) patients treated by submucosal diathermy would undergo this procedure again.

Discussion

For reduction of the lower turbinates different operative methods are used [5, 15–18]. This reflects the unsatisfactory therapeutic situation. Disadvantages of conventional techniques are tendency for postoperative hemorrhages, damage of the mucous membranes which is significant for some procedures, and limited long-term success [9, 15, 19]. Advantages of the laser surgical procedures are the reduced rates of postoperative hemorrhages, the limited tissue damage and the good long-term results [10, 16, 20]. A careful application is the requirement for a successful laser-surgical treatment of enlarged turbinates. To be eligible for laser surgery the nasal obstruction must be caused mainly by swelling or hypertrophy of the mucous membranes [9, 21–23].

Several, widely used procedures have been described in the literature, where the CO_2 laser is used. Selkin [12] uses the CO_2 laser for resection of the mucous membrane on the turbinates with the laser power set at 15–18 W. Elwany and Harrison [16] vaporize the mucous membranes in the anterior one-third with a laser power of 20–30 W. Fukutake et al. [9] remove the whole mucous membrane of the inferior turbinate by vaporisation with 20–25 W once a week for 5 weeks.

We use a different technique: single laser spots (power density: 2,038 W/cm^2; application duration 1 s) are applied in the anterior part of the lower turbinate. This induces shrinking of the mucosa with subsequent scarring. Since enough intact mucous membrane remains, a sufficient reepithelisation is possible [21, 24]. This avoids excessive scarring. It also reduces incrustation which has been described by other authors and is most probably caused by an inappropriate high laser power and the resulting damage to the mucous membranes [9, 12, 25, 26].

Long-term results are most important to evaluate new operative procedures. We therefore prospectively studied the postoperative course for a minimum of 2 years and compared the results with patients treated by submucosal diathermy who were examined retrospectively.

Besides a reduced rate of postoperative complications laser surgery also has a better long-term outcome when compared to submucosal diathermy. The long-term success is due to the increased scarring of the mucous membranes of the anterior turbinate after laser therapy. More laser surgically treated patients would agree to another procedure when compared to patients treated by submucosal diathermy. This can be explained by higher effectivity and good results but also by a low rate of complications and an uncomplicated procedure which allows fast and pain-free treatment in an outpatient setting. Less postoperative wound care is necessary.

References

1   Mittelman H: CO$_2$-laser turbinectomies for chronic, obstructive rhinitis. Lasers Surg Med 1982;2:29–36.
2   Fanous N: Anterior turbinectomy. A new surgical approach to turbinate hypertrophy: A review of 220 cases. Arch Otolaryngol Head Neck Surg 1986;112:850–852.
3   Mabry RL: Inferior Turbinplasty: Patient selection, technique, and long-term consequences. Otolaryngol Head Neck Surg 1987;98:60–66.

4   Principato JJ: Chronic vasomotor rhinitis: Cryogenic and other surgical modes of treatment. Laryngoscope 1979;89:619–638.

5   Mabry RL: Surgery of the inferior turbinates: How much and when? Otolaryngol Head Neck Surg 1984;92:571–576.

6   Ohyama M, Yamashita K, Furuta S, Nobori T, Daikuzono N: Applications of the Nd:YAG laser in otorhinolaryngology; in Joffe SN, Oguro Y (eds): Advances in Nd:YAG Laser Surgery. Springer, Berlin, 1988, pp 156–165.

7   Moore JRM, Bicknell PG: A comparison of cryosurgery and submucous diathermy in vasomotor rhinitis. J Laryngol Otol 1980;94:1411–1413.

8   Devergan BK, Leach W: Submucosal diathermy of inferior turbinates. Eye Ear Nose Throat Mon 1976;55:156–159.

9   Fukutake T, Kumazawa T, Nakamura A: Laser surgery for allergic rhinitis. AORN J 1987;46: 756–761.

10 Lenz H: Acht Jahre Laserchirurgie an den unteren Nasenmuscheln bei Rhinopathia vasomotorica in Form der Laserstrichkarbonisation. HNO 1985;33:422–425.

11 Lippert BM, Werner JA, Hoffmann P, Rudert H: CO_2- und Nd:YAG-Laser: Vergleich zweier Verfahren zur Nasenmuschelreduktion. Arch Otorhinolaryngol 1992;(suppl II):116–117.

12 Selkin SG: Laser turbinectomy as an adjunct to septorhinoplasty. Arch Otolaryngol 1985;111: 446–449.

13 Werner JA, Lippert BM, Rudert H: Endoskopische Lasertherapie obstruktiver Atemwegserkrankungen; in Ginsbach G (ed): Verhandlungsbericht der Deutschen Gesellschaft für Lasermedizin e.V. Aachen, Ginsbach, 1992, pp 452–465.

14 von Haacke NP, Hardcastle PF: Submucosal diathermy of the inferior turbinate and the congested nose. ORL J Otorhinolaryngol Relat Spec 1985;47:189–193.

15 Warwick-Brown NP, Marks NJ: Turbinate surgery: How effective is it? A long-term assessment. ORL J Otorhinolaryngol Relat Spec 1987;49:314–320.

16 Elwany S, Harrison R: Inferior turbinectomy: Comparison of four techniques. J Laryngol Otol 1990;104:206–209.

17 Simpson GT, Shapshay SM, Vaughan CW: Rhinologic laser surgery. Otolaryngol Clin North Am 1983;16:829–837.

18 Werner JA, Rudert H: Der Einsatz des Nd:YAG-Lasers in der Hals-Nasen-Ohrenheilkunde. HNO 1992;40:248–258.

19 Jones AS, Lancer JM: Does submucosal diathermy to the inferior turbinates reduce nasal resistance to airflow in the long term. J Laryngol Otol 1987;101:448–451.

20 Levine HL: Lasers and endoscopic rhinologic surgery. Otolaryngol Clin North Am 1989;22: 739–748.

21 Hoffmann JF, Parkin JL: Rhinologic applications of laser surgery. Otolaryngol Clin North Am 1990;23:19–28.

22 Johnson LP: Nasal and paranasal sinus applications of lasers; in Davis RK (ed): Lasers in Otolaryngology: Head and Neck Surgery. Philadelphia, Saunders, 1990, pp 145–155.

23 Selkin SG: Pitfalls in intranasal laser surgery and how to avoid them. Arch Otolaryngol Head Neck Surg 1986;112:285–289.

24 Levine HL: The potassium-titanyl phosphate laser for treatment of turbinate dysfunction. Otolaryngol Head Neck Surg 1990;104:247–251.

25 Kawamura S, Fukutake T, Kubo N, Yamahita T, Kumazawa T: Subjective results of laser surgery for allergic rhinitis. Acta Otolaryngol (Stockh) 1993;500(suppl):109–112.

26 Werner JA, Rudert H: CO_2- und Nd:YAG-Laser: Beschreibung und Vergleich ihres Wirkungsgrades am biologischen Gewebe. Arch Otorhinolaryngol 1989;(suppl II):214–215.

Dr. B.M. Lippert, Department of Otorhinolaryngology, Head and Neck Surgery,
University of Kiel, Arnold-Heller-Strasse 14, D–24105 Kiel (Germany)

Rudert H, Werner JA (eds): Lasers in Otorhinolaryngology, and in Head and Neck Surgery.
Adv Otorhinolaryngol. Basel, Karger, 1995, vol 49, pp 122–124

....

Endoscopic Surgery of the Nose and Paranasal Sinuses with the Aid of the Holmium:YAG Laser

Jens Feyh

Klinik und Poliklinik für Hals-, Nasen-, Ohrenheilkunde, Klinikum Grosshadern,
München, Deutschland

Endoscopic sinus surgery has proved to be an effective technique for the treatment of sinusitis and nasal obstruction due to enlarged turbinates refractory to medical therapy. Although the endoscopic instrumentation provides excellent visualisation within the nasal cavity, bleeding during the operation still occurs and nasal packings have to be inserted following surgery. As an alternative endoscopic sinus and turbinate surgery, a holmium:YAG laser system was tested in patients with chronic obstruction of the nose due to enlarged middle and lower turbinates and in surgery of the infundibulum.

Method

A holmium:YAG laser system (Versa Pulse 2.1, Coherent) was used as light source delivering a 2,100-nm laser beam through a 50-μm quartz fiber. A specially designed hand piece with a 30° tip (Versatile®) served as beam applicator. The power settings were as follows: 8 pulses/s, average power 4.8 W; 0.6 J. Twenty-eight patients with the following disorders were treated with the hol:YAG laser: enlarged turbinates, 11; obstructed infundibulum, 11; nasal papilloma, 2; nasopharynx papilloma, 1; nasal synechia, 3.

Local anesthesia was conducted with cotton gauze strips inserted into the nasal cavity (pantocaine 8% and adrenaline).

The endoscopic operation was performed with a 30° endoscope (Karl Storz).

Results

With the laser, it was very simple to remove tissue from the enlarged turbinates and to separate synechias. No bleeding or pain occurred during the operation. In addition to the surgery focused on soft tissue, the shape of the middle turbinate (concha bullosa) was also changed by removing the lateral bony part. During and following the operation no edema or swelling of the turninates occurred and the patients were constantly asked about nasal obstruction relief.

In patients with chronic sinusitis due to obstruction of the infundibulum, the bulla ethmoidalis and cells of the ethmoid were opened as well as the maxillary sinuses. Limitations of the laser operations in the area of the agger nasi and uncinate process were due to bone heating. Power settings above an average of 4.8 W at 8 Hz applied to bony structures were painful.

After the operation no nasal packings were inserted and the patients were treated on an outpatient basis.

Wound healing was completed in 6–8 weeks following endoscopic surgery.

Discussion

The mode of action of the holmium:YAG laser as a high-energy pulsed laser system is based on nonlinear processes of photoablation, first described by Srinivasan and Mayne-Banton [1] in 1982. Laser pulses with power densities of 0.1–10 J/cm^2 are applied to the tissue in a nanosecond range. Thus, ablation of bone is possible at temperatures of 30–70 °C.

With increasing power densities tissue can be ionized leading to plasma free of electrons and finally to an optical shockwave. Furthermore, the different absorption characteristics of tissues do not affect the maintenance of the 'plasma cutting' [2, 3].

According to its special physical characteristics, the holmium:YAG laser can be used for endonasal surgery of the nose and paranasal sinuses.

Oswal and Bingham [4] described the successful laser treatment of turbinate hyperplasia with local anesthetics on an outpatient basis. They ablated the hyperplastic mucosa of the turbinates without observing postoperative swelling.

Woog et al. [5] used the holmium:YAG laser in one case of dacryocystorhinostomy with an endonasal approach with good results. The author emphasized the easy dissection of the anterior part of the middle turbinates on a nontouch mode. Thus, the risk of skull-base injuries by mechanical dislocation of the base of the middle turbinate is reduced significantly.

Further applications of this laser system may be in the field of ethmoid surgery, since the holmium:YAG laser is able to ablate mucosa and thin bone easily with good hemostasis.

References

1 Srinivasan R, Mayne-Banton V: Self-developing photoetchning of poly (ethylene terephthalate) films by far ultraviolet excimer laser radiation. Appl Phys Lett 1982;41:576.
2 Kautzky M, Susani M, Leukauf M, Schenk P: Holmium:YAG- und Erbium: YAG-Infrarotlaser-Osteotomie. Langenbecks Arch Chir 1992;377:300–304.
3 Kautzky M, Susani M, Schenk P: Holmium:YAG Infrarot Laser- und UV-Excimer. Laser-Effekte auf orale Schleimhautgewebe. Laryngorhinootologie 1992;71:347–352.
4 Oswal VH, Bingham BJG: A pilot study of the holmium YAG laser in nasal turbinate and tonsil surgery. J Clin Laser Med Surg 1992;37:65–68.
5 Woog JJ, Metson R, Puliafito C: Dacryocystorhinostomy with the Holmium:YAG Laser. Coherent. Company information.

Jens Feyh, MD, Klinik und Poliklinik für Hals-, Nasen-, Ohrenheilkunde,
Klinikum Grosshadern, Marchioninistrasse 15, D–81377 München (Germany)

Rudert H, Werner JA (eds): Lasers in Otorhinolaryngology, and in Head and Neck Surgery.
Adv Otorhinolaryngol. Basel, Karger, 1995, vol 49, pp 125–129

....

Histological Evaluation of Leukoplakia following CO_2 Laser Excision

A Clinical and Experimental Study

Bernd Fleiner [a], *Thomas Plath* [b]

[a] Department of Oral and Maxillofacial Surgery (Head: Prof. *F. Härle*),
University Hospital Kiel, and
[b] Department of Oral and Maxillofacial Surgery, Plastic Surgery
(Head: Prof. *B. Hoffmeister*), University Hospital Steglitz, Berlin, Germany

Exact histological examination of oral leukoplakia is of great clinical importance. Conventional surgical excision by scalpel is increasingly being replaced by carbon dioxide laser treatment [1–4]. The disadvantage of CO_2 laser therapy by vaporization of the whole lesion is that conventional biopsies are necessary in advance. On the other hand, it is possible to excise the whole lesion using a focused CO_2 laser as a cutting instrument [5–7]. This technique yields specimens from the whole lesion and permits a complete histological examination. The purpose of this study is to evaluate the influence of laser-induced thermic damage on the light-microscopic examination of these specimens.

A clinical and experimental study was performed to examine the influence of thermic damage caused by different laser power and laser techniques (continuous wave vs. pulsed wave) on histological examination.

Materials and Method

Clinical Study

Of 62 leukoplakia specimens excised from the floor of the mouth, the tongue and the cheek, 25 were randomly selected for retrospective analysis. All excisions had been performed with a CO_2 laser (medilas 1025, Sharplan Co.) using a handpiece or micromanipulator under the microscope. The laser was focused on the tissue surface in a continuous-wave mode with an average power of 3–5 W. The specimens were mounted on a piece of cork with needles and, after fixation in formalin (4%), embedded in paraffin. The hematoxylin-eosin-stained microtome cuts were examined light microscopically. We evaluated to what extent the examination of the resection margins, the epithelial layer and the basal membrane was influenced by thermic damage.

Furthermore, the breadth of the thermically influenced zone was measured. The zone was defined as the area of more intensive HE staining.

Experimental Study

Fourteen rats were submitted to CO_2 laser excisions of the cheek and tongue mucosa. Three 5×5 mm areas were excised in each animal. The above laser technique was applied with power settings from 1 to 5 W. The mode applied for excisions was continuous wave in group A and pulsed (0.1 s) in group B.

The specimens obtained were divided into two parts: half were prepared for HE staining and the rest were quick-frozen in liquid nitrogen at –196 °C.

To detect ATPase, a thermolabile enzyme, which denaturates at 56–58 °C, the lead-salt method (modified by Losda et al. [8] after Wachstein and Meisel) was used. As a result, ATPase-positive areas appear brown to black in color. Those free of enzymatic reactivity appear white and can be differentiated by light microscopy.

Results

Clinical Study

The epithelial layer of all 25 patient specimens could be evaluated with regard to cell dysplasia and the basal membrane. There was no damage at the basal membrane, which made it impossible to detect any infiltration of the underlying tissues. At the resection margins, on the other hand, carbonization had caused severe cell damage. Coagulation of the cells caused a thread-like alteration of the nucleus and disruption of the basal membrane.

The quality of the evaluation of the different areas of the specimens was estimated as follows:

Epithelial dysplasia:	evaluation without limitation
Basal membrane:	evaluation without limitation
Margins of resection:	evaluation partially limited or no evaluation possible

Measured values from the zone of thermic damage – defined as the area of more intensive HE staining – ranged from 0.3 to 0.9 mm, with a median of 0.5 mm. All severe cell damages at the margins of the resection were within this zone.

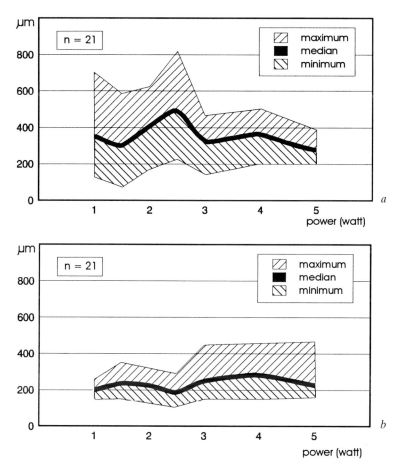

Fig. 1a, b. Medium, minimum and maximum of the breadth of the thermic damage of the continuous wave (*a*) and interval pulse (*b*) laser excision with different power settings (1–5 W).

Experimental Study

The excisions varied in thickness from 1.0 to 2.5 mm. The thermic damage at the resection margins did not differ from that in the patient specimens. Group A and group B were comparable with respect to the morphology of damaged tissue.

Measurement of the ATPase-negative zone revealed slight differences between the groups as well as between the different laser energies applied. The median of the ATPase-negative zone was about 200 μm in group B for all power levels from 1 to 5 W. Low-power excision (1–2.5 W) showed lower maxima (≤ 350 μm) than higher energies (≤ 500 μm). In group A, however, the

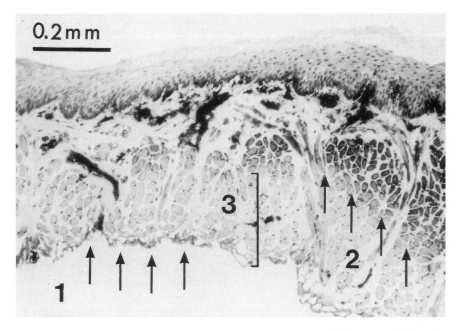

Fig. 2. Carbon dioxide laser excision of the lingual mucosa of a hamster. ATPase detection by peroxydase reaction. Coagulation effects at the margins of the resection (1). The border between ATPase reaction and ATPase-negative zone can be clearly identified (2). ATPase-negative zone (3).

median value varied between 250 and 500 µm, and the highest values of up to 800 µm (maxima) were found in low-power excisions (1–2.5 W) (fig.1 a, b).

It should be noted that the ATPase-negative zone is not identical to the light-microscopically identified zone of cellular damage caused by carbonization. The carbonization effects were within the zone smaller than 100 µm (fig. 2).

Discussion

Following laser excision of oral leukoplakia [1, 9, 10], the complete specimens can be examined and the thermic damage does not interfere with the light-microscopic examination, except for the carbonization effect at the resection margin. Comparison of the HE-stained specimens from the patients and the animal model discloses similar thermic effects on the cellular and acellular substances. The thermic influence on ATPase detection by the lead-salt reaction leads to a sharp discrimination of the thermic influence zone. It can be shown that the zone of direct cell carbonization and coagulation is always within the ATPase-negative zone, which can thus be regarded as the area of thermic tissue damage, even if enzymohistochemical methods are applied.

Quantitative measurements of thermic damage show that no advantage can be gained by applying very low energies of 1–2.5 W. Focused application of CO_2 laser at average power of 3–5 W is recommended for the excision of oral leukoplakias. In this power range the modes of application – continuous wave or pulsed – have no significant influence on the amount of thermic damage to the specimens.

The results of the study confirm our opinion that carbon dioxide laser excision is the method of choice in the therapy of oral leukoplakia. Keeping a safety distance of 1 mm at the resection margins, the histological examination is not influenced. Preoperative biopsies are not necessary, because the complete lesion can be excised without discomfort to the patient. The technique of vaporization, which involves no clinical advantage and does not permit histological examination, should no longer be performed.

References

1   Dunsche A, Kreusch TH, Sauer M: Die Leukoplakie der Mundschleimhaut – eine retrospektive Studie an 161 Patienten. Dtsch Zahnärztl Z 1992;47:869–871.
2   Gerlach KL, Roodenburg JLN, Herzog M, Horch H-H, Panders AK, Pape H-D, de la Coix WF, Vermey A: Die Therapie oraler Präkanzerosen mit dem CO_2-Laser – Langzeitergebnisse aus drei Kliniken. Dtsch Zahnärztl Z 1993;48:48–50.
3   Horch H-H, Gerlach KL, Schaefer HE, Pape H-D: Erfahrungen mit der Laserbehandlung oberflächlicher Mundschleimhauterkrankungen. Dtsch Z Mund Kiefer Gesichts Chir 1983;7: 31–35.
4   Roodenburg JLN, Panders AK, Vermey A: Carbon dioxide laser surgery of oral leukoplakia. Oral Surg Oral Med Oral Pathol 1991;71:670–674.
5   Chiesa F, Tradati N, Sala L, Costa L, Podrecca St, Boracchi P, Bandieramonte G, Mauri M, Molinari R: Follow-up of oral leukoplakia after carbon dioxide laser surgery. Arch Otolaryngol Head Neck Surg 1990;116:177–180.
6   Fleiner B, Lüttges J, Hoffmeister B: Histologische Beurteilbarkeit von Mundschleimhautveränderungen nach CO_2-Laserresektion. Dtsch Zahnärztl Z 1993;48:53–55.
7   Frame JW: Removal of oral soft tissue pathology with the CO_2-laser. J Oral Maxillofac Surg 1985;43:850–855.
8   Losda Z, Grossran R, Schiebler TH: Enzymhistochemische Methoden. Heidelberg, Springer, 1976.
9   Guerry TL, Silverman S Jr, Dedo HH: Carbon dioxide laser resection of superficial oral carcinoma: Indications, techniques and results. Ann Otol Rhinol 1986;95:547–555.
10 Luomanen M: Experience with a carbon dioxide laser for removal of benign oral soft-tissue lesions. Proc Finn Dent Soc 1992;88:49–55.

Bernd Fleiner, DMD, MD, Department of Oral and Maxillofacial Surgery,
University Hospital Kiel, Arnold-Heller-Strasse 16, D–24105 Kiel (Germany)

Rudert H, Werner JA (eds): Lasers in Otorhinolaryngology, and in Head and Neck Surgery.
Adv Otorhinolaryngol. Basel, Karger, 1995, vol 49, pp 130–131

....

Laser Surgery in Lingual Tonsil Hyperplasia

Jos J.M. van Overbeek, Jurgen P. te Rijdt

Department of Otorhinolaryngology, Martini Hospital, Groningen,
The Netherlands

From 1982 to 1992, 76 patients with hyperplastic lingual tonsils were treated with CO_2 laser surgery. Table 1 gives some characteristics of the series. The CO_2 laser proved to be successful and has become our first choice of therapy. Under general anesthesia, with nasotracheal intubation, the lingual tonsil is broadly visualized with an endoscope which has been specially developed (Medin, Groningen, the Netherlands) for this purpose [1]. With a CO_2 laser in combination with an operating microscope and micromanipulator, the lymphoid humps are excised, mostly in one session. Persistent bleeding can be stopped by electrocoagulation with an insulated forceps or suction tube.

It is important to reserve surgical therapy only for good indications (table 2). Recurrent lingual tonsillitis can be regarded as the best indication. In all other cases a careful decision has to be made. Mild complaints do not need more than mild therapy, and when neurotic elements are suspected, surgery should be avoided.

Results

The CO_2 laser therapy was very well tolerated and characterized by the near absence of postoperative edema.

The results in the patients with recurrent tonsillitis were superior to those in the patients with globus feelings (table 3).

Though preoperative bleeding could always be controlled by coagulation, we were confronted with a postoperative hemorrhage 4 times, in one case with a fatal course.

Table 1. Laser surgery in lingual tonsil hyperplasia (characteristics of series)		
Period	1983–1992
Number of patients	76
Total number of treatments	96
Age	15–72 years (mean 38)
Sex	56 females, 20 males

Table 2. Indications for laser surgery in lingual tonsil hyperplasia (n = 76)

	n	%
Tonsillitis	46	61
Globus	22	29
Snoring, cough, etc.	8	11

Table 3. Results and complications after laser surgery in lingual tonsil hyperplasia

	Tonsillitis (n = 46) %	Globus (n = 22) %
Good	41	35
Relief of symptoms	46	45
No relief	13	20

Complications in 96 treatments: postoperative hemorrhage 4%, mortality 1%.

Conclusions

We conclude that the CO_2 laser and a special endoscope are the tools of choice for surgery of lingual tonsil hyperplasia. The success rate is strongly dependent on the diagnostic criteria for its application. The procedure can be difficult and complicated by the risk of severe postoperative hemorrhage.

Reference

1 Wouters B, van Overbeek JJM, Buiter CT, Hoeksema PE: Laser surgery in lingual tonsil hyperplasia. Clin Otolaryngol 1989;14:291–296.

Jos J. M. van Overbeek, Department of Otorhinolaryngology, Martini Hospital, NL–9700 RM Groningen (The Netherlands)

Rudert H, Werner JA (eds): Lasers in Otorhinolaryngology, and in Head and Neck Surgery.
Adv Otorhinolaryngol. Basel, Karger, 1995, vol 49, pp 132–135

....

CO$_2$ Laser Surgery for Benign Tumors of the Oral Cavity

Rudolf Grossenbacher

Department of Otorhinolaryngology, Head and Neck Surgery, Kantonsspital,
St. Gallen, Switzerland

Surgery with the CO$_2$ laser beam was introduced into clinical medicine some 20 years ago. Soon, benign and malignant changes in the oral cavity were excised using the CO$_2$ laser. The advantages of surgery with the CO$_2$ laser, such as reduced bleeding in the area undergoing surgery, a relatively slight degree of postoperative edema, only minor postoperative pain, made it appear to be an advantageous instrument in the treatment of such alterations in the oral cavity as well. With the further development of the optical system for the CO$_2$ laser with corresponding reduction of the spot size, the indications have become more solid because, particularly with the smaller focus, mucous membrane alterations across a wide area can be removed from the remaining oral mucosa very accurately. The use of the CO$_2$ laser beam in the high-energy pulse form (superpulse), which is possibly of advantage for other indications, has not proven to be of significant advantage in the oral cavity, a fact which we have been able to show in an experimental study [1]. For this reason, at St. Gallen's ENT department, the CO$_2$ laser beam is nowadays used as continuous wave for the removal of benign tumors or mucosal alterations in the oral cavity either directly with a hand piece or by way of a micromanipulator with the aid of the operational microscope.

Material and Methods

Between 1978 and 1993, a total of 132 benign alterations and tumors of the oral cavity have been treated with the CO$_2$ laser beam. The accurate breakdown of the corresponding diagnoses is listed in table 1. We initially used the Coherent System 400 CO$_2$ surgical laser system, and from 1985 onwards, the Cooper Model 2502 CO$_2$ laser system,

Table 1. CO_2 laser surgery for 132 benign tumors of the oral cavity (1978–1993)

Leukoplakia	35	Lichen ruber erosivus	5
Fibroma	25	Granular cell tumors	2
Ranula	16	Lymphangioma	2
Papilloma	14	Monomorphic adenoma	1
Hemangioma	13	Neurofibroma	1
Granuloma	9	Lipoma	1
Pleomorphic adenoma	7	Neuroma	1

which has the facility for both microspot and hand-piece application. Depending on size, localization and type of pathological lesions to be treated, the operation was performed under local anesthesia or under nasotracheal intubation anesthesia. Basically, the pathological change in the tissue was entirely excised and subsequently subjected to histological examination. Tissue removal by vaporization was performed only in rare cases in which the benign nature of the lesion was clear. The wounds were not closed but always left to heal by secondary intent.

Results

The 132 patients (77 males, 55 females) were aged between 2 and 70 years.

All the benign lesions were removed by laser surgery in each case without complications and subsequent healing left only a fine scar, which did not produce any functional disorder in any of the patients. Six of the 35 patients with leukoplakia developed a recurrence, which was again excised by laser in 3 patients, while the other 3 patients have simply been kept under regular observation. Treatment of the ranula was carried out by means of total excision of the inner mucosal lining of the ranula as well and not merely with a usual marsupialization in order to prevent the possible development of a recurrence. In our group, we have not seen any recurrences. Hemangiomas could also be removed – partly with the aid of bipolar coagulation in the case of larger bleeding vessels – entirely and without complications with the aid of the CO_2 laser, although in the treatment of hemangiomas, the CO_2 laser does not supply the ideal wavelength. Teleangiectatic granulomas with a high tendency to relapse (fig. 1, 2) have also been recurrence free to date after total CO_2 laser excision.

The field of vision was good in all operations carried out on patients when using the CO_2 laser. Larger arterial branches of the lingual artery or the greater palatine vessel had to be bipolarly electrocoagulated or suture stitched. The surface of the wound is left, as previously mentioned, to heal by secondary

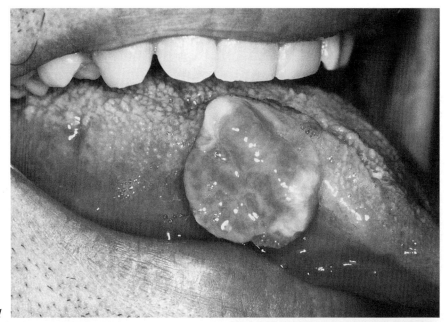

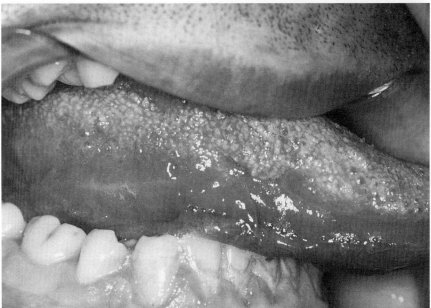

Fig. 1. Teleangiectatic granuloma of the right tongue, recurrence after conventional excision.

Fig. 2. Same patient, situation 6 months after laser excision of the teleangiectatic granuloma. Soft scar, no functional loss, no further recurrence.

intent. None of the patients suffered from breathing difficulties. The majority of patients showed only minor discomfort following laser surgery. Food was already being taken through the mouth on the first day following surgery. The duration of wound healing was directly correlated to the surface of the wound and lasted between 3 and 7 weeks. Scars were noticeably soft in nearly all patients, and in no case was mouth function impaired to any significant degree.

Discussion

The advantage of using the CO_2 laser in treating pathological changes of the mucous membrane of the oral cavity is that an optimal field of vision over the area undergoing surgery is guaranteed by the fact that there is no or very little bleeding during surgery. When a surgical microscope is also used, this enables pathologically altered tissue to be extirpated with a great degree of accuracy and minimum functional disorder. Moreover, surgery can be undertaken on patients with blood-clotting disorders with a minimum risk of hemorrhage.

A further advantage of laser surgery, in our view, is the slight degree of postoperative edema, together with either a frequent absence or only a slight degree of pain. Moreover, scar formation is, for the most part, soft following CO_2 laser surgery, so that functional impediments are rarely expected.

To sum up, we can state that by using the CO_2 laser beam, the removal of easily accessible tumors or mucous membrance alterations in the oral cavity can be performed with few complications and only minor patient discomfort.

Reference

1   Grossenbacher R, Sutter R: Carbon-dioxide laser surgery in otorhinolaryngology: Pulsed beam versus continuous wave beam. Ann Otol Rhinol Laryngol 1988;97:222–228.

Prof. R. Grossenbacher, Department of Otorhinolaryngology, Head and Neck Surgery, Kantonsspital, CH–9007 St. Gallen (Switzerland)

Rudert H, Werner JA (eds): Lasers in Otorhinolaryngology, and in Head and Neck Surgery.
Adv Otorhinolaryngol. Basel, Karger, 1995, vol 49, pp 136–139

....

Use of Carbon Dioxide Laser in the Therapy of Benign Oral Soft-Tissue Lesions

Anton Dunsche[a], *Bernd Fleiner*[a], *Hendrik Terheyden*[a], *Bodo Hoffmeister*[b]

[a] Department of Oral and Maxillofacial Surgery (Head: Prof. F. Härle),
University Hospital Kiel, and
[b] Department of Oral and Maxillofacial Surgery (Head: Prof. B. Hoffmeister),
University Hospital Steglitz, Freie Universität Berlin, Germany

Since 1991, our department has used the carbon dioxide laser for removal of oral soft tissue pathologies. 161 operations were performed on 115 patients. 197 lesions were removed. 25% were oral cancer, 75% were benign. Distribution of the most frequent pathologies is listed in table 1.

Precancerous Lesions

Previous studies have shown malignant transformation of oral leukoplakia in 0.3–18.0% [1–3]. Our treatment protocol until 1991 required excision of precancerous lesions showing signs of moderate or severe dysplasia. Dispite this fact our patients (n = 161), which were followed up from 1980 until 1991 showed malignant transformation in 6.2%. Malignant transformation was also seen in leukoplakias without dysplasia [4].

Therefore, we recommended that each leukoplakia which does not disappear after elimination of etiological factors should be completely removed [4].

From 1991 until 1994, 95 precancerous lesions (88 leukoplakias, 5 erythroplakias and 2 lichen planus) were removed using the carbon dioxide laser. 62 of them were localized in the floor of the mouth and on the tongue, both high-risk localizations for malignant transformation [1–4]. By power setting from 3 to 5 W, we most commonly use the carbon dioxide laser in focussed mode for excision of the lesions. In most cases, a micromanipulator was used under the microscope [5, 6]. All specimens were investigated histologically. In cases of leukoplakia, epithelial dysplasia and basement membrane could be investi-

Table 1. Treated benign lesions (n = 149)

Precancerous lesions	95
– Leukoplakia	88
– Erythroplakia	5
– Lichen planus	2
Persistent mucoceles and ranulas	7
Gingival hyperplasias	10
Denture-induced hyperplasias	6
Other benign lesions	31

gated as well as the resection margins [7]. Functional results are good. Wound healing took 2–4 weeks. Postoperatively, no infection occurred during the wound-healing period. Postoperative bleeding occurred in one case. While dissecting the salivary duct (n = 13) during partial resection from the floor of the mouth stenosis with subsequent sialoadenitis occurred in 7 cases. Marsupialisation should therefore be carried out.

Five lesions clinically regarded as precancer already showed early cancer histologically. Five of 95 lesions (5.9%) showed local recurrence during the first year of follow-up. Further follow-up is necessary. After surgical excision, a recurrence rate of 20% up to 35% is estimated [8, 9]. Carbon dioxide laser vaporization shows recurrence in 14.2%, but in only 10% of the cases using the microscope [10]. Frame [6] noticed recurrences in 8% after carbon dioxide laser excision.

Persistent Mucoceles or Ranulas

Persistent mucoceles or ranulas were treated in 7 cases. The thin cystic sac of ranulas is opened at its widest circumference. The upper part is resected and the bottom is left open. The procedure is relatively bloodless with good visualization especially on the floor of the mouth. We did not see a recurrence in any of the 5 cases (fig. 1). Mucoceles were completely removed together with the associated minor salivary gland.

Drug-Induced Gingival Overgrowth

In 5 patients during 10 sessions, the overgrowth was removed epiperiostally by power setting from 3 to 8 W. Vaporization and resection is combined to prevent injury of the periosteum and dental hard tissue. Radical resection

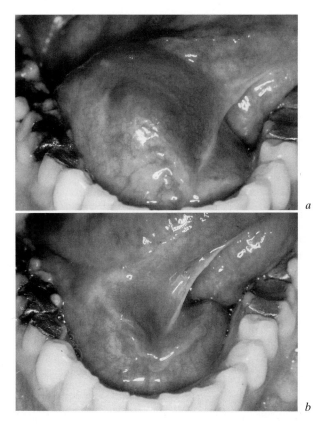

Fig. 1.a Recurrent ranula which has been operated twice. *b* Sixteen months after treatment by CO_2 laser without stenoses of the salivary duct or recurrence.

and optimal postoperative oral hygiene are necessary for the prevention of recurrence. In 1 patient, the periosteum was injured, which caused no further problem. The technique is difficult and the operating time is relatively long.

Denture-Induced Hyperplasia

Newtons type III, granular inflammation or inflammatory papillary hyperplasia, is induced by trauma from ill-fitting dentures and promoted by candida infection. It has to be removed if it persists after antifungal therapy. We use the carbon dioxide laser for excision up to the periosteum, without damaging it. Other denture-induced hyperplasias like fibromas, especially when situated in the sulcus, can be completely excised with only little scarring or distortion of the soft tissues [6].

Carbon dioxide laser excision is a useful supplement in surgery of benign oral mucosal lesions. In contrast to vaporization, histological examination is possible and should be done in all precancerous lesions. Due to the relatively low rate of recurrences and good functional results, it is the treatment of choice for oral leukoplakias especially when localized on the floor of the mouth or on the tongue.

References

1 Gupta PC, Metha FS, Daftary DK, Pindborg JJ, Bhonsle PN, Jalnawalla PN, Sinor PN, Pitkar VK, Murti PR, Irani RR, Shah HT, Kadam PM, Iyer KSS, Hegde AK, Chandrasheka GK, Shroff BC, Sahiar BE, Metha MN: Incidence rates of oral cancer and natural history of oral precancerous lesions in a 10 year follow-up study of Indian villagers. Commun Dent Oral Epidemiol 1980;8:287–333.
2 Silverman S, Gorsky M, Lozada F: Oral leukoplakia and malignant transformation. Cancer 1984;53:563–568.
3 Lind PO: Malignant transformation in oral leukoplakia. Scand J Dent Res 1987;95:449–455.
4 Dunsche A, Kreusch TH, Sauer M: Die Leukoplakie der Mundschleimhaut – eine retrospektive Studie an 161 Patienten. Dtsch Zahnärztl Z 1992;47:869–871.
5 Chiesa F, Tradati N, Sala L, Costa L, Podrecca ST, Boracchi P, Bandieramonte G, Mauri M, Molinari R: Follow-up of oral leukoplakia after carbon dioxide laser surgery. Arch Otolaryngol Head Neck Surg 1990;116:177–180.
6 Frame JW: Removal of oral soft tissue pathology with the CO_2 laser. J Oral Maxillofac Surg 1985;43:850–855.
7 Fleiner B, Lüttges I, Hoffmeister B: Histologische Beurteilbarkeit von Mundschleimhautveränderungen nach CO_2-Laserresektion. Dtsch Zahnärztl Z 1993;48:53–55.
8 Vedtofte P, Holmstrup P, Hörting-Hansen E, Pindborg JJ: Surgical treatment of premalignant lesions of the oral mucosa. Int J Oral Maxillofac Surg 1987;16:656–664.
9 Mincer HH, Coleman SA, Hopkins KP: Observations on the clinical characteristics of oral lesions showing histological epithelial dysplasia. Oral Surg 1972;33:389–399.
10 Gerlach KL, Pape H-D, de Lacroix WF, Roodenburg JLN, Panders AK, Herzog M, Horch H-H: Die Therapie oraler Präkanzerosen mit dem CO_2-Laser – Langzeitergebnisse aus drei Kliniken. Dtsch Zahnärztl Z 1993;48:48–50.

Dr. Dr. Anton Dunsche, Department of Oral and Maxillofacial Surgery, University Hospital, Arnold-Heller-Strasse 16, D–24105 Kiel (Germany)

Rudert H, Werner JA (eds): Lasers in Otorhinolaryngology, and in Head and Neck Surgery.
Adv Otorhinolaryngol. Basel, Karger, 1995, vol 49, pp 140–143

....

Microendoscopic CO$_2$ Laser Surgery of the Hypopharyngeal (Zenker's) Diverticulum

Jos J.M. van Overbeek

Department of Otorhinolaryngology, Martini Hospital, Groningen, The Netherlands

All the 545 patients included in this report, except for 1 of the 2 patients with a carcinoma of the pouch, were treated endoscopically at the ENT Departments of the University Hospital and the Martini Hospital, Groningen, The Netherlands, from 1964 until 1992. Eleven of the patients experienced a recurrent diverticulum after previous surgical diverticulectomy elsewhere (table 1). We began to treat Zenker's diverticula endoscopically [1] using the procedure described by Dohlman and Mattson [2]. With the increase in the number of patients, the technique and instruments used have been improved [3]. In 1981, we started to apply a microendoscopic laser procedure with a specially designed double-lipped endoscope (Medin, Groningen, The Netherlands), the operating microscope, and the CO$_2$ laser. The microscope affords an excellent view of the bridge to be divided. For the technique of microendoscopic surgery, general anesthesia is necessary, but when there is a contraindication to general anesthesia, endoscopic surgery may be performed under local anesthesia with the Dohlman electrocoagulation technique. In microendoscopic surgery, very precise division of the tissue bridge is possible. The nature of the tissues in the plane of division can be observed by the magnification of the microscope. The wound edges separate immediately, resulting in a wedge-shaped excision. This separation is caused by the severed cricopharyngeal muscle fibers from the upper esophageal sphincter, which are readily identifiable. The CO$_2$ laser has poor coagulation capacities, and, therefore, bleeding sometimes must be controlled with brief electrocoagulation using an insulated microsurgical forceps or suction tube. After the operation, all patients were given antibiotics and liquid food for 1 week. Swallowing liquids was nearly always possible, and a feeding tube was therefore seldom used. Barium radio-

Table 1. Some characteristics of a series of 545 patients with a hypopharyngeal (Zenker's) diverticulum

Mean age, years	67.1
Over 90 years	13
Male/female ratio	1.5:1
Race	white
Recurrence after external operation	11
Carcinoma in the pouch	2
Familial occurrence (4 families)	9
Small diverticula (<1 vertebral body)	51
Medium-sized diverticula	384
Large diverticula (>3 vertebral bodies)	110

Table 2. Results after endoscopic treatment of 544 patients with a hypopharyngeal (Zenker's) diverticulum

Results	n	%
Very satisfied	493	90.6
Fairly satisfied	47	8.6
Not satisfied	4	0.7

graphy was performed 5 days and 6 weeks after the endoscopic treatment. Even those patients in whom there was radiologic evidence of a residual diverticulum were usually free of symptoms. The information obtained with radiography should not be overestimated, and repetition of endoscopic treatment after 6 weeks was only carried out if the patient had residual symptoms. In patients with very large diverticula, we preferred to divide the spur in two or three sessions.

Results

For the 544 patients treated endoscopically between 1964 and 1992, the follow-up is at least 10 months. Of the patients, 493 are very satisfied (90.6%) and 47 (8.6%) are fairly satisfied with the results obtained (table 2). Although one patient died of cardiac failure 2 days postoperatively, the complications we observed were mostly not serious and our complication rate was very low

Table 3. Complications after endoscopic treatment of 544 patients with a hypopharyngeal (Zenker's) diverticulum

Complication[1]		Comments
Endoscopic electrocoagulation technique (n = 328)		
Death	1	2 days postoperatively of cardiac failure
Mediastinitis	7	6 cured by conservative therapy, 1 mediastinotomy
Hemorrhage	4	endoscopically controlled by electrocoagulation
Esophagotracheal fistula	1	closed spontaneously within 3 weeks
Emphysema	10	only temporary in the neck
Tendency to stenosis	8	satisfactory results following endoscopic dilations
Microendoscopic CO_2 laser treatment (n = 216)		
Death	–	
Mediastinitis	5	3 cured by conservative therapy, 2 by mediastinotomy
Hemorrhage	1	packing during 24 h
Esophagotracheal fistula	–	
Emphysema	7	only temporary in the neck
Tendency to stenosis	–	

[1] More than one complication occurred in 4 patients.

(table 3). Our experience indicates that the risk of mediastinitis is smaller than often suggested in the presence of adhesions between diverticulum and the posterior esophageal wall. When comparing the coagulation technique and laser technique, we noticed that patients treated with the CO_2 laser experienced less pain during the first postoperative day and consequently took food more readily. Radiologic follow-up revealed no essential difference in the final results between the patients treated with the electrocoagulation technique or with the CO_2 laser. In our laser-treated patients, however, we have not noticed a tendency to stenosis, which has been seen in 8 patients treated with the electrocoagulation technique.

Conclusions

Our results obtained over many years with endoscopic treatment of Zenker's diverticulum have prompted us to continue to use this approach and to further perfect the techniques involved [4]. Exposure of the tissue bridge between esophagus and diverticulum, with the aid of the specially designed double-lipped scope, poses no significant problems. The use of the operating microscope and the CO_2 laser makes this technique an improvement on the original Dohlman's method. Very precise severance of the spur is feasible. The magnification makes it possible to identify the nature of the tissue in the plane of severance and to follow the separation of the muscle fibers. Hemorrhage, if it occurs, can be arrested with insulated microsurgical instruments without causing more than minimal tissue damage. With severance of the tissue bridge between esophagus and diverticulum, a transmucosal upper esophageal sphincterotomy is achieved and an ample overflow from diverticulum to esophagus is effected in a very short operation time.

It is somewhat surprising that endoscopic treatment of the hypopharyngeal diverticulum has failed to become more popular. An important advantage of endoscopic management is that it can be carried out in patients whose general condition is poor. The procedure requires experience, but we believe experience is likewise important in the transcutaneous approach.

In view of our results in 545 patients, we feel justified in maintaining that endoscopic surgical treatment of Zenker's diverticulum can be regarded as a safe and effective method of treatment. The risk of complications with this method is minimal with our technique as described.

References

1   Van Overbeek JJM, Hoeksema PE: Endoscopic treatment of the hypopharyngeal diverticulum: 211 cases. Laryngoscope 1982;92:88–91.
2   Dohlman G, Mattson O: The endoscopic operation for hypopharyngeal diverticula. Arch Otolaryngol 1960;71:744–752.
3   Van Overbeek JJM, Hoeksema PE, Edens ETh: Micro-endoscopic surgery of the hypopharyngeal diverticulum using electrocoagulation or carbon dioxide laser. Ann Otol Rhinol Laryngol 1984;93:34–36.
4   Van Overbeek JJM: Meditation on the pathogenesis of hypopharyngeal (Zenker's) diverticulum and a report of endoscopic treatment in 545 patients. Ann Otol Rhinol Laryngol 1994;103:178–185.

Jos J.M. van Overbeek, Department of Otorhinolaryngology, Martini Hospital,
NL–9700 RM Groningen (The Netherlands)

Rudert H, Werner JA (eds): Lasers in Otorhinolaryngology, and in Head and Neck Surgery.
Adv Otorhinolaryngol. Basel, Karger, 1995, vol 49, pp 144–147

....

Endoscopic Laser Myotomy in Cricopharyngeal Achalasia

C. Herberhold, E.K. Walther

Department of Otorhinolaryngology, University of Bonn, Germany

Dysfunction of the pharyngoesophageal junction is a rare condition and may cause severe signs and symptoms of dysphagia. The underlying abnormality is a dysfunction of the cricopharyngeal muscle. Patients with a prominent cricopharyngeal bar visible on radiography are generally considered to have spasms of the cricopharyngeus, which is the major muscle component of the upper esophageal sphincter (UES). This condition has been termed 'cricopharyngeal achalasia' [1]. The pathophysiology may be a lack of or incomplete relaxation of the UES during deglutition [2, 3]. An increase in intrabolus pressure may preserve normal transsphincteric flow rates even though the UES does not open normally. More recent manometric investigations showed, however, that UES relaxation itself is not necessarily impaired [1]. This may explain why the detection of dyskinetic UES action does not always cause dysphagia [4]. In those cases, an incoordination between relaxation in relation to pharyngeal contractions can be detected.

A primary form of cricopharyngeal achalasia is separated from a secondary form in the course of neuromuscular disorders or local lesions such as pharyngeal tumors, postsurgical scarring with pharyngoesophageal stenosis, congenital disorders or external compression of the pharyngeal wall. Different therapeutic principles are known. Medical treatment is recommended only in cases of secondary achalasia depending on the basic disease such as thyroid-dysfunction-associated myopathy, Parkinson's disease, or myasthenia gravis [3, 5]. Balloon dilatation has not proved effective in the long run despite some promising early reports [6]. More reasonable are surgical procedures employing extramucous myotomy of the cricopharyngeus muscle [7–9]. Since microendoscopic surgery of hypopharyngeal diverticulas has proved beneficial

[10–12], we undertook to evaluate laser endoscopic myotomy of the cricopharyngeus muscle in achalasia without external approach.

Patients and Diagnosis

Thirty-two patients with cricopharyngeal achalasia were included in the study. Additionally, 7 of those patients had also developed hypopharyngeal diverticulum and in 5 patients pharyngoesophageal stenosis due to scarring was evident. The mean age of the patients (15 male, 17 female) was 60.3 years with 2 children younger than 1 year. All patients had a history of dysphagia for solid food on an average of 14 months. The etiology of the achalasia was in 14 cases of primary (idiopathic) origin and in 18 cases secondary to pharyngolaryngeal tumor therapy (n = 12), strumectomy (n = 2), or neurogenous disorders (n = 4).

Preoperative diagnosis is based upon history and clinical and radiological examination as well as pharyngoesophageal computer manometry. Fluoroscopy reveals a dorsally located cricopharyngeal muscle bulge associated with a total or near total impression of the pharyngoesophageal bolus. On computer manometry, a high-pressure zone in the pharyngoesophageal segment with failing or prolonged relaxation and incoordination to deglutition is detected [13]. The prestenotic pressure rise may be responsible for the development of hypopharyngeal diverticula [14]. If individually necessary, imaging for detection of aberrant vascularisation (i.e. following thyroidectomy, dysontogenetically with innominate artery) is employed. As there is a known association with cricopharyngeal achalasia [15], gastroesophageal reflux has to be excluded prior to surgery.

Technical Management and Equipment

In the meantime, the surgical procedure has been well established in our department. We use a common CO_2 laser with a regular rigid laser esophagoscope. The endoscope is attached to the operating microscope with a conventional 350- to 400-mm objective to visualize the prominent cricopharyngeus. Standard laser safety precautions are taken including a smoke evacuator channel in the endoscope. In general, the laser radiation output used lay between 5 and 20 W with a focused or slightly defocused beam. The total average time of laser radiation was 131 s.

Once the endoscope has been positioned properly, the hypertrophic cricopharyngeus bulge impedes further passage into the esophagus. Aberrant blood vessels present with transmitted pulsation. The transverse muscle bulge is then gradually dissected in a vertical direction exactly in the median plane with repeated pushing and pulling the endoscope back and forth. The proceeding myotomy is indicated visually through the operating microscope by lateral retraction of the divided muscle fibers resulting in a wedge-shaped excision. A 'last' layer of muscle fibers is left. Bleeding of the tissue is minimal and easily controlled with electrocautery. The surgical procedure usually takes only a few minutes. Postoperatively, the patients are monitored carefully for fever, chest pain, tachycardia, and subcutaneous emphysema. Antibiotic cover is limited to a perioperative prophylaxis with administration of broad-spectrum antibiotics. Clear liquids and noncorpuscular diets can be given immediately followed by a soft diet. A control fluoroscopy after 1 week is recommended. Patients can usually be discharged after 2 days.

Results

The postoperative complication rate is low. Twenty-seven of 32 patients had a normal postoperative course without any pathological events. Three patients had a transitory gastric tube for several days. Two patients developed postoperative complications. In one case prolonged intubation was necessary due to a transient supraglottic edema and in the other an imminent mediastinitis had to be suspected by clinical symptoms, which was surgically revised by lateral cervicotomy without finding a mediastinal leakage. Postoperative hemorrhage was not noticed in any case.

In the observation period of up to 7 years, an improvement of oral food intake was evident in all cases but one. One female patient did not show any improvement and later underwent myofascial flap reconstruction of the pharyngoesophageal segment.

Seven patients showed some residual fluoroscopic evidence of former achalasia with neither dysphagia nor impairment of oral intake of solid food. Four patients had to undergo one to three repeat endoscopic procedures before the resolution of symptoms. Twenty-four of 32 patients showed normal clinical and radiological conditions.

Conclusion

From the results presented, it can be concluded that laser myotomy is an appropriate procedure in the surgical treatment of cricopharyngeal achalasia. Performing laser myotomy, it is important to do a step-by-step dissection of the cricopharyngeus muscle with a remaining 'last' layer of muscle fibers. The indication is secure once gastroesophageal reflux conditions are excluded or eliminated.

References

1   Dantas RO, Cook IJ, Dodds WJ, Kern MK, Lang IM, Brasseur JG: Biomechanics of cricopharyngeal bars. Gastroenterology 1990;99:1269–1274.
2   Ekberg O, Wahlgren L: Dysfunction of the pharyngeal swallowing. A cineradiographic investigation of 854 dysphagial patients. Acta Radiol 1985;26:389–395.
3   Kreitner KF, Teifke A, Staritz M, Heintz A: Zur Röntgenologie und Klinik der krikopharyngealen Achalasie. Röntgen-Bl 1990;43:89–93.
4   Cook IJ: Cricopharyngeal function and dysfunction. Dysphagia 1993;8.244–251.
5   Hurwitz AL, Duranceau A: Upper esophageal sphincter dysfunction. Pathogenesis and treatment. Am J Dig Dis 1978;23:275.
6   Mihailovic T, Perisic VN: Balloon dilatation of cricopharyngeal achalasia. Pediatr Radiol 1992;22:522–524.

7   Berg HM, Jacobs JB, Persky MS, Cohen NL: Cricopharyngeal myotomy: A review of surgical results in patients with cricopharyngeal achalasia of neurogenic origin. Laryngoscope 1985;95: 1337–1340.

8   Calcaterra TC, Kadell BM, Ward PH: Dysphagia secondary to cricopharyngeal muscle dysfunction. Surgical management. Arch Otolaryngol 1975;101:726–729.

9   McKenna JA, Dedo HH: Cricopharyngeal myotomy: Indications and technique. Ann Otol Rhinol Laryngol 1992;101:216–221.

10 Holinger LD, Benjamin B: New endoscope for (laser) endoscopic diverticulotomy. Ann Otol Rhinol Laryngol 1987;96:658–660.

11 Laubert A, Lehnhardt E: Die endoskopische Schwellenspaltung, eine Alternative bei der operativen Behandlung von Zenkerschen Divertikeln. HNO 1989;37:211–215.

12 van Overbeek JJM, Hoeksema PE, Edens ETh: Microendoscopic surgery of the hypopharyngeal diverticulum using electrocoagulation or carbon dioxide laser. Ann Otol Rhinol Laryngol 1984;93:34–36.

13 Walther EK, Herberhold C: Operative Therapie der Dysphagie bei amyotropher Lateralsklerose; in Dengler R, Zierz S, Jerusalem F (Hrsg): Amyotrophe Lateralsklerose. Stuttgart, Thieme, 1994.

14 Seaman WB: Pharyngeal and upper esophageal dysphagia. JAMA 1976;235:2643.

15 Henderson RD, Hanna WM, Henderson RF, Marryatt G: Myotomy for reflux-induced cricopharyngeal dysphagia: Five-year review. J Thorac Cardiovasc Surg 1989;98:428–433.

Eberhard K. Walther, MD, Universitäts-HNO-Klinik Bonn, Sigmund-Freud-Strasse 25, D–53105 Bonn (Germany)

Rudert H, Werner JA (eds): Lasers in Otorhinolaryngology, and in Head and Neck Surgery.
Adv Otorhinolaryngol. Basel, Karger, 1995, vol 49, pp 148–152

....

Laser Lithotripsy of Salivary Duct Stones

H. Iro, J. Zenk, W. Benzel

Department of Oto-Rhino-Laryngology, Head and Neck Surgery
(Head: Prof. *M. E. Wigand*), University of Erlangen-Nuremberg, Germany

Besides piezoelectric extracorporeal lithotripsy of salivary stones [1], there are different possibilities for intracorporeal, endoscopically guided lithotripsy when treating sialolithiasis. Because of the specific anatomy of the peripheral salivary ducts and due to the very often bright color of the salivary stones, several systems are not suitable for clinical management as proved experimentally in in vitro and in vivo studies.

Because of the severe tissue damage shown in animal experiments, the use of electrohydraulic intracorporeal lithotripsy as well as Excimer laser lithotripsy seems not to be justified for treating human sialolithiasis despite the good stone fragmentation in vitro [2, 3]. The Nd:YAG laser and the Alexandrit laser were not suitable in in vitro studies due to the insufficient fragmentation of salivary calculi [2]. On the contrary, with the help of a Rhodamine 6-G flashlamp pumped dye laser (Lithognost, Telemit Co., Germany), a sufficient stone fragmentation rate of 75% was achieved in vitro. With this dye laser an integrated stone-tissue detection system on the basis of fluorescence spectroscopy is connectable. While activating this stone-tissue detection system in animal experiments no tissue damage was detected in the peripheral salivary ducts of rabbits during shockwave application. Because of these experimental results this dye-laser system seems to be suitable for use in human sialolithiasis [4]. In the following, we report our clinical experiences using the Rhodamine 6-G dye laser in the intracorporeal endoscopically guided treatment of salivary calculi of the submandibular gland.

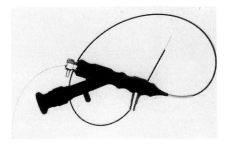

Fig. 1. Endoscope with the laser fibre inserted.

Material and Methods

Patients

Only patients with symptomatic solitary submandibular stones situated near the hilus were eligible for this prospective study.

All together, 8 women and 12 men aged between 34 and 55 years were included. The sizes of the salivary calculi were seen on ultrasound, and concrements larger than 10 mm were excluded from the study. Patients suffering from salivary calculi of the parotid gland were also excluded, as for sufficient insertion of the endoscope into the salivary duct slitting of the duct about 2 weeks before laser treatment is necessary. Slitting of the parotid salivary duct has a high risk of obstruction due to scarring and stenosis.

Endoscope

We used a flexible endoscope with an outer diameter of 1.6 mm and a working channel of 600 µm both for endoscopic diagnosis as well as for intracorporeal guided laser lithotripsy. This endoscope, which is only available as a prototype, can actively be bent along one level (fig. 1).

Lithotripter

The Rhodamine 6-G dye laser which we used for our studies emits at a wave-length of 595 nm with a maximum pulse energy of 120 mJ.

Energy is transmitted through extremely thin, flexible glass fibres with a diameter of 250 µm. Laser pulses are applied to the stone in a noncontact mode. A connectable automatic feedback cut-out (stone-tissue detection system) regulates the intensity of the laser beam. The preset level of energy is only applied if the beam of light is reflected from the surface of the stone. If the beam makes contact with tissue, the energy level of the laser pulse is automatically reduced to approximately 10% of its original energy by means of fluorescence spectroscopy after about 200 ns.

Application of Intracorporeal Laser Lithotripsy

Two weeks after slitting and marsupialisation of the duct of the submandibular gland intracorporeal endoscopically guided laser lithotripsy was performed. After local anesthesia, the endoscope was inserted into the duct until the salivary stone was localized. After-

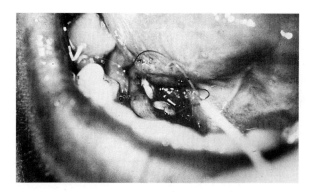

Fig. 2. Removal of fragments by a dormia basket after laser lithotripsy of a submandibular gland stone.

wards, the laser fibre together with the irrigation unit were put into the working channel of the endoscope. The treatment of salivary calculi with laser pulses happened under direct optical control with simultaneous NaCl irrigation.

With the option 'stone tissue detection activated', up to 1,500 pulses were applied to the concrement with maximum energy. In those cases where complete fragmentation of the stone was achieved, treatment was stopped before completing the 1,500 impulses. After laser lithotripsy, fragments had been extracted with the help of dormia baskets (fig. 2). Moreover, patients were asked to enforce saliva secretion (lemon juice, chewing gum) in order to reach an expulsion of the fragments through the salivary duct.

Follow-Up Period

Each patient was controlled sonographically and clinically at least 6 months after laser lithotripsy. Attention was especially directed to the rate of stone-free patients as well as to the rate of patients free of any discomfort.

Results

Only 2 of 20 salivary calculi (10%) were destroyed completely. Among these, patients lacking concrements were evaluated clinically and sonographically 6 months after laser lithotripsy. Eleven stones (55%) were only partly fragmented. In these cases, parts of the concrements were still detectable, but more or less significantly reduced in size. In the follow-up period, 8 of these 11 patients' felt completely free of discomfort. Three of them further reported transient swelling of the salivary gland at meals. In 7 patients (35%), laser lithotripsy was not successful at all, no calculus reaction towards the laser beams was detected. These patients' symptoms of obstructive sialadenitis were unchanged. Thus, treatment of submandibular gland calculi smaller than 10 mm resulted in a 10% rate concerning complete disappearance of concrements and a 50% rate of no further discomfort caused by sialolithiasis. Stones which showed any reaction to the laser beams were commonly dark in color, whereas concrements which showed no reaction were brightly colored, meaning that a major part of the laser light was reflected.

Discussion

Treatment of ureteral calculi and concrements within the descending ducts of the gallbladder by means of intracorporeal laser lithotripsy has already been established clinically.

Concerning the intracorporeal laser lithotripsy of salivary calculi, until now only clinical experiences made by an Excimer laser system have been published [5, 6]. In the course of in vitro and animal experiment studies, it has been demonstrated that application of laser pulses created by an Excimer laser lead to severe damage of the salivary duct as well as important surrounding structures (vessels, nerves) [2, 5]. Moreover, no results concerning the stone-free rate after Excimer-laser lithotripsy are known.

With regard to in vitro and animal experiment studies, the Rhodamine 6-G dye laser seems to be usable even in the narrow peripheral salivary ducts of humans [4].

For introduction of the endoscope, a slitting of the salivary duct of the afflicted gland is necessary, especially in the area of the orifice, as the most narrow parts of the ducts are localized there. Because of the particular preference concerning stenosis of Stensens duct after slitting it, removal of parotid calculi by intracorporeal laser lithotripsy does not seem to be suitable.

We have not seen such stenosis after slitting of Whartons duct in our clinical experience nor have such events been reported in literature. Therefore, endoscopically guided, intracorporeal laser lithotripsy is well suited to remove concrements of the submandibular gland.

During the follow-up period, our results with intracorporeal, endoscopically guided laser lithotripsy showed a free-of-stone rate of only 10% but a distinctly higher rate of 50% concerning complete loss of discomfort.

As a result of our experiences, intracorporeal, endoscopically guided laser lithotripsy – we therefore used a dye laser system with connectable automatic feedback cut-out – can be recommended only in a restricted manner as an alternative to other already established methods of treatment in human sialolithiasis (extracorporeal piezoelectric shockwave lithotripsy, sialodochoplasty, submandibulectomy).

The clinical use of intracorporeal, endoscopically guided lithotripsy with a dye laser should be reserved for special cases.

Nevertheless, in these singular cases complete loss of salivary calculi can be obtained and loss of any complaints can be achieved in a larger number of patients.

References

1   Iro H, Schneider HTh, Födra C, Waitz G, Nitsche N, Heinritz HH, Benninger J, Ell Ch: Shock-wave lithotripsy of salivary duct stones. Lancet 1992;339:1333.
2   Iro H, Zenk J, Benzel W, Hosemann WG, Hochberger J, Ell Ch: Experimentelle Untersuchungen zur Laser-Lithotripsie von Speichelsteinen. Lasermedizin 1992;8:110.
3   Zenk J, Benzel W, Hosemann WG, Iro H: Experimental research on electrohydraulic lithotripsy of sialolithiasis. Eur Arch Otorhinolaryngol 1992;249:436.
4   Benzel W, Hofer M, Hosemann WG, Iro H: Laser-induced shock wave lithotripsy of salivary calculi with automatic feedback cessation in case of tissue contact: in vitro and animal experiments. Eur Arch Otorhinolaryngol 1992;249:437.
5   Gundlach P, Scherer H, Hopf J, Leege N, Müller G: Die endoskopisch kontrollierte Laserlithotripsie von Speichelsteinen: In-vitro-Untersuchungen und erster klinischer Einsatz. HNO 1990; 38:247.
6   Königsberger R, Feyh J, Goetz A, Schilling V, Kastenbauer E: Die endoskopisch kontrollierte Laserlithotripsie zur Behandlung der Sialolithiasis. Laryngol Rhinol Otol 1990;69:322.

Priv.-Doz. Dr. H. Iro, Department of Oto-Rhino-Laryngology, Head and Neck Surgery, Waldstrasse 1, D–91054 Erlangen (Germany)

Rudert H, Werner JA (eds): Lasers in Otorhinolaryngology, and in Head and Neck Surgery.
Adv Otorhinolaryngol. Basel, Karger, 1995, vol 49, pp 153–157

....

Experiences with Laser Surgery in Benign and Malignant Findings of the Oro- and Hypopharynx

Reinhard G. Matschke

Klinik für Hals-, Nasen-, Ohrenkrankheiten, Kopf- und Halschirurgie der
Ruhr-Universität Bochum, Prosper-Hospital Recklinghausen, Deutschland

It was only 30 years ago that Patel [1] described continuous-wave laser action on vibrational-rotational transitions of CO_2 and the most promising was the one with a length of 10.6 μm. It was only some years later that the power of the carbon dioxide lasers could be raised by the addition of nitrogen and helium. Today, the carbon dioxide laser is one of the most powerful continuous-wave lasers and has within one decade become a well-accepted surgical tool.

In otorhinolaryngology, the CO_2 laser has become well accepted especially for surgical procedures in tissues which are strongly supplied with blood vessels. During the past years there have been several indications for surgical therapy in the oropharynx and hypopharynx in benign and malignant findings which called for laser treatment because of the outstanding option of reduced bleeding, e.g. hyperplasia of the lingual tonsils, hypopharyngeal diverticula, and oropharyngeal scars after tumor surgery. The aim of this study was to demonstrate some experiences with this kind of laser therapy.

Method and Material

During the period 1989 to 1994, we performed 97 operations with the carbon dioxide laser on 76 patients with benign and malignant findings in the oro- and hypopharynx. Gender distribution was equal: 38 females and 38 males. The mean age was 48.7 years, the youngest patient being 1 year old and the oldest 88.

Totally, 56 operations of the lingual tonsil were done including 4 cases with malignant lymphoma. Dissections of diverticula in the hypopharynx and the upper esophagus were performed 14 times, debulking of a tumor and/or dissection of scars was necessary

12 times. We removed juvenile papilloma of the hypopharynx and larynx 7 times, cysts of the soft palate and hemangioma of the tongue floor were removed 5 times. We tried to resect the vocal cord 3 times because of palsy of the n. laryngeus recurrens. Most of the operations were lingual tonsillotomies (58%) because of hyperplasia and recurrent tonsillitis.

Complaints before surgery were dominated by dysphagia. Other complaints were pain in the throat, dyspnea, foreign body feeling, hoarseness, regurgitation, and snoring. After surgery, swallowing pain lasting nearly 2 weeks was described by most of the patients. In 5 cases, these complaints lasted longer than 14 days and were experienced as a burden.

Results

Generally, surgery was tolerated without major problems. Nevertheless, we had to face some complications. After laser surgery, we observed recurrence, bleeding, and delayed wound healing. Recurrence after resection of a hyperplastic lingual tonsil occurred 6 times and demanded surgery again. After resection of malignant lymphoma of the lingual tonsil we observed early bleeding (case 4). In 4 cases we saw an extremely delayed wound healing with severe perichondritis. The total rate of complications of the retrospectively evaluated 97 operations was 28%. Without considering the palliative operations in which recurrences have to be expected per se, the complication rates are still relatively high!

The overall time of clinical treatment after all operations lasted 7.2 days (SD 5.6 days). Considering the lingual tonsillotomies (58%) only, the time of hospital treatment was 5.5 days. Thus, the average stay in hospital after tonsillectomy by conventional surgery, which is 5.2 days in our clinic, is not delayed essentially.

Excerpted Case Reports

Case 1
W.S., a 56-year-old male patient, complained of dysphagia and sometimes hoarseness of the voice for several months. During otorhinolaryngological examination, a hyperplasia of the lingual tonsil was found which displaced the epiglottis in a way that the evaluation of the larynx was not possible. No other pathological findings could be found. An adenotonsillectomy had been performed during childhood. A microlaryngoscopy under general anesthesia was combined with laser tonsillotomy of the lingual tonsil. From the right vocal cord, a small tumor was removed which was diagnosed histologically as a fibroepithelioma. The postoperative history was uneventful. Four weeks later, the patient again complained of dysphagia and massive granulative tissue was found in the tongue floor region. The resection of hyperplastic tonsillar tissue and granulative tissue was again

performed by laser surgery under general anesthesia and the postoperative history was again uneventful. Three years later, the patient suffered from dysphagia and swallowing pain again, and the tongue floor was enlarged and showed inflammation. After conservative treatment with antibiotics and decongestants without success, another resection of lingual tonsillar tissue was performed. The histological diagnosis again came out with chronic tonsillitis and fibrotic peritonsillitis. After an uneventful postoperative history, the patient is now free of disease and has no complaints. Voice function is not disturbed and the microlaryngoscopic findings are satisfactory.

Case 2
M.M., a 9-year-old boy, suffered from juvenile papillomatosis of the larynx since his 4th year of life. He had already experienced several operations to secure the airway after severe hypopnea. A therapeutic experiment with α-interferon had not led to a status free of disease. Former resections of the papillomata had been performed conventionally with surgical instruments. When he was referred to our clinic, the papillomatous tissue had spread even to the hypopharynx. First laser resection showed good results but had to be repeated already 5 months later without reaching the spread-out of the former status. A third resection was necessary only 26 months later. This time the papillomatous tissue was localized solely to the inner larynx. Traumatization of the larynx after the laser therapy was reduced drastically, tracheostomy was not necessary. The voice function of the child is now delightfully good. The histological diagnosis confirmed the clinical findings.

Case 3
Because of a laryngeal cancer, laryngectomy with neck dissection had to be performed in 59-year-old T. H. Histological evaluation of the specimen confirmed resection borders free of tumor and no disease of the lymph nodes. The postoperative history was uneventful, but 3 months after surgery the patient complained of dysphagia. Otorhino-laryngological examination revealed a very small scarred shrinkage in the hypopharynx, which was resected under general anesthesia with a CO_2 laser. Histologically, there was no recurrence of the malignant disease. Only 4 months later, the patient complained of the same difficulties and showed the same findings. Again, the scar was resected with the laser and again recurrence of the malignant disease was excluded histologically. The postoperative history was uneventful and the patient free of complaints after the healing of the wound. Another 3 months later, the complaints of dysphagia and regurgitation occurred again, and the patient presented the same findings in the hypopharynx. Resection of the scar tissue and histological evaluation excluded malignant recurrence. This time the patient received psychotherapy and the fear or recurrence could be taken from him. After an uneventful postoperative healing period, the patient is now free of complaints for 4 years and we could not find any more scarring shrinkage during the regular follow-up examinations.

Case 4
K.O., a 79-year-old female patient, suffered from chronic lymphocytic leukemia with monstrous infiltrations of the lingual tonsil and the adenoids which had been diagnosed 2 years previously. This caused strong dysphagia, blocked nose, heavy snoring, and dry mouth. Therapy with a cytostatic agent had not reduced the infiltrations and the patient's

complaints persisted. Nonetheless, because of the risk of bleeding, the internal specialist advised against surgical therapy. But symptoms grew worse and the general condition of the patient deteriorated. To secure the airway, the hyperplastic lingual tonsils were resected by means of a carbon dioxide laser and the final hemostasis was performed with a neodym-YAG laser. Nevertheless, 2 h after surgery, there was bleeding again which made surgical hemostasis necessary again with the neodym-YAG laser because the sutures had failed. Postoperatively, a massive leukocytosis occurred which could be controlled with chlorambucil (Leukeran®). Infiltrations of the lingual tonsils turned out histologically as a non-Hodgkin's lymphoma of lower malignancy. Because of the large wound, the reduction of the adenoidal infiltration was postponed and the patient recovered slowly. Dysphagia vanished but she still had a blocked nose. The patient postponed further surgery, and died 1 year later of the lymphoma.

Conclusions

Diseases of the lingual tonsil are very rarely reported either in clinical practice or in the literature [2]. It is stated that practitioners very often ignore this part of the pharynx in their diagnostic and differential-diagnostic efforts [3, 4]. Nevertheless, chronic inflammation of the lingual tonsil can be the source of manifold complaints like sore throat, pain, dysphagia, foreign body feeling, hoarseness, and hacking cough. After surgery of malignant tumors of the mouth floor or the larynx, e.g. laryngectomy, patients sometimes complain of dysphagia due to scars or diverticula of the hypopharynx. The carbon dioxide laser was used by many surgeons for more than 20 years to resect benign and malignant tumors of the oral cavity and hypopharynx [5–8] with good success. Especially in tissues with strong blood supply could we confirm in our 5 years' experience that surgery was made possible by the CO_2 laser. Nevertheless, surgery with the laser turned out to be not without complications. Complications after surgery mainly consisted of recurrence, bleeding and delayed wound healing. The rate of bleeding was 11 % in laser lingual tonsillotomy, which is a little higher than following conventional tonsillectomy [9, 10]. The rate of recurrence correlates with the incidence of 'recurrence' of blocked nose after adenotomy. To reduce the rate of recurrence after lingual tonsillotomy the resection should be radical enough. The occurrence of scars and strictures in the oro- and hypopharynx is often observed after radical tumor surgery. They may lead to manifold complaints including dysphagia and swallowing pain. Thus, the quality of life of the patient is often drastically reduced. These scars can be treated functionally with good effect. Sometimes it happens in patients after laryngectomy that the substitutional voice of the esophagus is diminished temporarily. Histological evaluation of a specimen of the resected tissue is always necessary because of the possibility of recurrence.

The most impressive case of delayed wound healing occurred after resection of a vocal cord because of bilateral nerve palsy in a patient which had been irradiated 17 years earlier because of a thyroid carcinoma. The wound healing was disturbed in a way that led to a perichondritis which ran out of control and demanded laryngectomy in the end.

Nonetheless, in well-selected cases the success of laser surgery in otorhinolaryngology cannot be reached with another method and has proved to be an indispensable tool in our clinic.

References

1   Patel CKN: Continuous-wave laser action on vibrational-rotational transitions of CO_2. Phys Rev 1964;136:1187.
2   Krespi YP: Laser lingual tonsillectomy. Laryngoscope 1989;99:131–135.
3   Cohen HB: The lingual tonsil: General consideration and its neglect. Laryngoscope 1917;27:691–700.
4   Joseph M, Reardon E, Goodman M: Lingual tonsillectomy: A treatment for inflammatory lesions of the lingual tonsil. Laryngoscope 1984;94:179–184.
5   Strong MS, Vaughan CW, Jako GJ, Polanyi T: Transoral resection of cancer in the oral cavity: The role of CO_2 laser. Otolaryngol Clin North Am 1979;12:207–214.
6   Steiner W, Jaumann MP, Wigand ME: Laserendoskopie in Pharynx, Larynx und Trachea. Arch Otorhinolaryngol 1980;227:586–594.
7   McDonald GA, Simpson GT: Transoral resection of lesions of the oral cavity with the carbon dioxide laser. Otolaryngol Clin North Am 1983;16:839–847.
8   Grossenbacher R: Laserchirurgie in der Oto-Rhino-Laryngologie; in Becker W, Boenninghaus H-G, Naumann HH (Hrsg): Aktuelle Oto-Rhino-Laryngologie, Heft 9. Stuttgart, Thieme, 1985, pp 52–67.
9   Matschke RG, Plath P, Wierich W: Der Peritonsillarabszess. Z Allg Med 1987;63:339–344.
10 Brauneis J, Wittich I, Laskawi R: Ist die Tonsillektomie bei peritonsillärem Abszeß noch zeitgemäß? Otorhinolaryngol Nova 1993;3:200–203.

Priv.-Doz. Dr. Reinhard G. Matschke, Klinik für Hals-, Nasen-, Ohrenkrankheiten, Kopf- und Halschirurgie im Klinikum Schwerin, Wismarsche Strasse 397, D–19049 Schwerin (Germany)

Rudert H, Werner JA (eds): Lasers in Otorhinolaryngology, and in Head and Neck Surgery.
Adv Otorhinolaryngol. Basel, Karger, 1995, vol 49, pp 158–161

....

CO$_2$ Laser Surgery for Benign Lesions of the Vocal Cords

Rudolf Grossenbacher

Department of Otorhinolaryngology, Head and Neck Surgery,
Kantonsspital St. Gallen, Switzerland

The most significant progress in CO$_2$ laser surgery since its introduction to clinical medicine 20 years ago was the possibility of the reduction of the spot size to approximately 0.25–0.3 mm with the aid of the micromanipulator. Thanks to this microspot, surgery of the endolarynx can now be performed with the aid of the surgical microscope with a focal length of 400 mm, thus ensuring a high degree of accuracy. Due to the reduction of the spot size, the energy density can be increased (square function); in other words, the exposure time of the CO$_2$ laser beam in the tissue is reduced and thus the corresponding carbonization changes decrease which proves to be advantageous particularly for the removal of smaller benign vocal cord alterations which for the most part are not very rich in vascularization.

Material and Methods

During the period from 1978 through 1993 we have treated benign alterations of the vocal cords with the CO$_2$ laser beam. The individual indications and diagnoses are listed in table 1. The operations were all performed in insufflation anesthesia on the relaxed patient, initially with the aid of an intubation tube packed in reflecting aluminum foil. Later on, the metal tube according to Norton was used, and for the last few years we have been using a fully flexible metal tube with an internal diameter of 5 mm. This tube was specially developed for jet ventilation. Thus, the endolarynx can be excellently adjusted, and due to its reduced diameter the tube does not have an impeding effect on the operating environment. Depending on the localization and type of the lesion to be removed, the adjacent endolaryngeal areas are protected by moist pads against any unintentional laser beam effect.

Table 1. CO₂ laser surgery for benign lesions of the vocal cords

Polyps	Hemangioma
Reinke edema	Obstructive scars
Granuloma	Bilateral vocal cord
Papilloma	palsy
Cysts	Glottic sulcus
Nodules	Tuberculosis
Hyperkeratotic lesions	Amyloid tumor

Results

The most frequent indication for CO_2 laser application was voice-impairing polyps which could be removed without any complications. Furthermore, bilateral polypoid degeneration (Reinke edema) was treated with the CO_2 laser. Since the microspot has been available, the mucous membrane is lifted – whenever possible – only by separating a flap over the polypoid degeneration; the pathological substance is then removed submucosally, partly with the suction tip, partly – in case of adherent, highly viscous alterations – vaporized, and the mucous membrane flap is folded back over the free vocal cord edge. An additional excellent indication for the CO_2 laser in benign vocal cord alterations are the recurrent granulomas of the vocal cord and at the arytenoid cartilage developing after trauma, after intubation or voice overstrain. The teleangiectatic granulomas in this area, which have a high relapse tendency, could be accurately removed with the CO_2 laser, and the recurrence rate could be reduced very significantly as compared to conventional treatment. The same is true in the case of papilloma treatment with the CO_2 laser, although recurrences occur here as well; however, the recurrence interval appeared to be longer since the CO_2 laser beam was introduced. Moreover, the postoperative scar formation is rather slight. Submucous cysts can also be totally removed, and due to corresponding mucous membrane flaps the patient is able to speak again practically normally 1 or 2 days after surgery if the free vocal cord edge was left intact (fig. 1, 2). Vocal cord nodules can also be removed accurately with the microspot, and the same applies to the other indications listed in table 1. Glottic sulcus should be mentioned in particular. In 3 patients with such an alteration, we vaporized the epithelium in the glottic sulcus and left the wound to heal by secondary intent. The scar resulting in the healing phase filled the sulcus so that in these 3 cases a substantial improvement of the

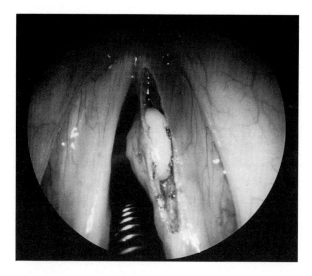

Fig. 1. Submucosal cyst of the right vocal cord after CO_2 laser microspot incision of the overlying mucosa.

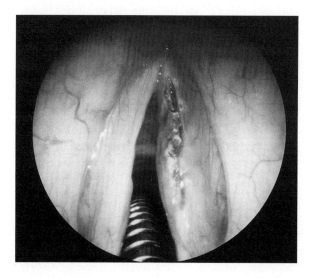

Fig. 2. The mucosal flap is repositioned on the vocal cord after total excision of the submucosal cyst. Good voice function the day following surgery.

voice quality was achieved. A rare indication nowadays is vocal cord tuberculosis, which, however, must be taken into consideration more frequently once again. The alterations within the framework of vocal cord tuberculosis, which in most cases are very similar to a carcinoma, are dealt with by excisional biopsy.

Discussion

The availability of the microspot (spot size 0.25–0.3 mm) resulted in a significant expansion of the indication spectrum in the field of endolaryngeal microscope-assisted surgery, and this both for benign and of course malignant alterations. Thanks to the microspot, mucous membrane flaps can actually be formed, which makes it possible to remove submucous alterations without putting too much strain on the normal mucous membrane and thus guaranteeing a rapid healing and excellent voice quality. In our opinion, special pathological alterations such as glottic sulcus, bilateral vocal cord paralyses, recurrent granulomas, etc., can be treated more rapidly with the CO_2 laser than by applying conventional procedures. The advantages such as excellent field of vision in the area undergoing surgery due to an absence or only slight degree of bleeding and particularly a slight degree of postoperative edema have been mentioned several times already, and they are very advantageous particularly in the case of endolaryngeal operations, since within the framework of the laser-surgical approach a tracheotomy never became necessary. For the future development, it would be very desirable if the beam diameter could be reduced once again by half in order to make yet finer and more precise incisions with the laser beam on the delicate, endolaryngeal structures. However, it can be assumed that this requirement will probably be better met in the future with lasers of a different wavelength.

Prof. Dr. R. Grossenbacher, Department of Otorhinolaryngology, Head and Neck Surgery, Kantonsspital, CH–9007 St. Gallen (Switzerland)

Rudert H, Werner JA (eds): Lasers in Otorhinolaryngology, and in Head and Neck Surgery.
Adv Otorhinolaryngol. Basel, Karger, 1995, vol 49, pp 162–165

....

Laser Surgery for Laryngeal Papillomatosis

Christoph G. Mahnke

Department of Otorhinolaryngology, Head and Neck Surgery,
University of Kiel, Germany

Laryngeal papillomatosis is a benign tumor disease induced by HPV 6 or 11. As of today no curative therapy is available. New therapeutic concepts have been reported and discussed controversely, most recently treatment with interferon or acyclovir or photodynamic therapy. These methods lack long-term results. They are also noncurative and have major side effects. Evaluation of new methods is difficult because of the long course of this disease. The symptomatic removal of papillomas is so far the only method where long-term results are available. Here the CO_2 laser and cold cutting instrument are the methods most commonly used. They will be compared.

Patients and Methods

The charts of all 95 patients who were treated for laryngeal papillomatosis at the Department of Otorhinolaryngology, University of Kiel between 1960 and 1990 were analyzed retrospectively. Fifty-three were male and 42 female. The following aspects were studied: age at first diagnosis, clinical course, form of therapy, recurrences and complications such as tracheostomy and glottic webs.

Before 1979, the main form of treatment was removal with cold cutting instrument or by cryosurgery. Since 1979 the CO_2 laser has been used for the treatment of laryngeal papillomatosis. It is used with the operating microscope and a modern micromanipulator (focus diameter 0.25 mm). The laser power is set between 1 and 2 W, correlating to a power density of 2,000–4,000 W/cm^2. This technique causes a precise cut with a reduced zone of carbonisation and minimal bleeding. In cases with defined histology the laser can also be used for vaporisation of the papillomas. If papillomas are found in the anterior commissure they are only removed on one side. The contralateral side is then cleared in a second operation 6 weeks later to avoid glottic webs.

During highly active phases of the disease (e.g. recurrences every 6 weeks or less) papillomas are removed to ensure safe airways and function of the vocal cords. Meticulous removal of all papillomas is done during phases of lower activity. This regimen avoids damage to the functional structures of the larynx.

Since the main form of therapy changed during the observation period, the patients can be divided into three groups (table 1): (a) patients treated with conventional surgery only; (b) patients treated by laser surgery only, and (c) patients with a prolonged course of the disease requiring surgery during both eras.

Results

At first diagnosis most patients were in their first or fourth decade. The sex destribution was equal. In 58% of the patients only one or two operative procedures were necessary. Analysis of the clinical course showed that puberty did not have any effect. Twenty-five patients were younger than 16 years at first diagnosis. In only 5 of these was the last recurrence observed between the ages of 10 and 20.

Table 1 shows the number of operations and complications for the three different groups. The rate of complications was much lower in the group of patients treated with the laser only.

In 4 patients subsequent malignancies developed.

Discussion

Epidemiology

Respiratory papillomatosis is a disease of all ages which is first diagnosed most commonly in the first or fourth decade. We did not find any changes in the clinical course during puberty. This has also been described by Lindeberg and Elbrond [1]. The term recurrent respiratory papillomatosis does therefore appear more appropriate than juvenile or adult laryngeal papillomatosis.

The malignant transformation is a well-known problem. The rate of 4.2% observed in this study corresponds to earlier reports [2, 3]. It underlines the need for repeated histological examination of the specimen and allows vaporisation of the lesions only in cases with certain histology.

Laser vs. Conventional Surgery

When discussing the surgical therapy one must keep in mind the systemic nature of this disease. Papillomavirus can be detected not only in the lesions but also in the intact mucous membranes all over the upper aerodigestive tract [4, 5]. For this reason surgery cannot be curative. The surgical removal of pa-

Table 1. Forms of therapy and complications

Form of therapy	Pa-tients n	Opera-tions n	Aver-age	Glottic webs	Tracheos-tomy
Conventional surgery only	40	97	2.4	10	4
Laser surgery only	30	101	3.3	1	0
Both methods	25	laser 88 conven-tional 72	6.4	4[1]	2[1]

[1] After conventional surgery.

pillomas must be limited to restore function of the larynx without causing further damage.

The use of the laser did not reduce the rate of recurrence. It did, however, cut back the rate of complications. The reduced number of glottic webs may be a result of the less traumatic technique when using the laser. The immediate hemostasic effect of the laser allows a better exposure with a more precise removal of the papillomas and less unintensional damage to the functional structures of the larynx. The use of the operating microscope further improves the exposure. The papillomatous lesions tend to bleed intensely when incised or even grasped only with conventional instruments. In some cases, it was impossible to remove all lesions with cold cutting instruments in one operation when bleeding developed so that repeated procedures a few days later or even tracheostomy were necessary.

Tracheostomy is regarded as contraindicated in this disease since it supports spread of the papillomas in the trachea which is a severe complication [6]. After the introduction of the CO_2 laser no tracheostomy was necessary.

Conclusion

Recurrent respiratory papillomatosis is a disease of all ages most commonly first diagnosed in the first or fourth decade. Puberty has no influence on the clinical course of this disease. At present, no curative therapy is available so that treatment has to be symptomatic. Here the CO_2 laser is the preferred method since it is less traumatic to the functional structures of the larynx and reduces the number of complications such as glottic webs and tracheostomy.

References

1 Lindeberg H, Elbrond O: Laryngeal papillomas: The epidemiology in a Danish subpopulation 1965–1984. Clin Otolaryngol 1990;15:125–131.
2 Lindeberg H: Laryngeal papillomas: Histomorphometric evaluation of multiple and solitary lesions. Clin Otolaryngol 1991;16:257–260.
3 Yoder MG, Batsakis JG: Squamous cell carcinoma in solitary laryngeal papilloma. Otolaryngol Head Neck Surg 1980;88:745–748.
4 Steinberg BM, Topp WC, Schneider PS, Abramson AL: Laryngeal papillomavirus infection during clinical remission. N Engl J Med 1983;308:1261–1264.
5 Ogura H, Watanabe S, Fukushima K, Baba Y, Masuda Y, Fujiwara T, Yabe Y: Persistence of human papillomavirus type 6e in adult multiple laryngeal papilloma and the counterpart false cord of an interferon-treated patient. Jpn J Clin Oncol 1993;23:130–133.
6 Cole RR, Myer CM, Cotton RT: Tracheotomy in children with recurrent respiratory papillomatosis. Head Neck 1989;11:226–230.

Dr. C.G. Mahnke, Department of Otorhinolaryngology, Head and Neck Surgery,
University of Kiel, Arnold-Heller-Strasse 14, D–24105 Kiel (Germany)

Rudert H, Werner JA (eds): Lasers in Otorhinolaryngology, and in Head and Neck Surgery.
Adv Otorhinolaryngol. Basel, Karger, 1995, vol 49, pp 166–169

....

Combined Laser Surgery and Adjuvant Intralesional Interferon Injection in Patients with Laryngotracheal Papillomatosis

C. Herberhold, E.K. Walther

Department of Otorhinolaryngology, University of Bonn, Germany

Since the discovery of a viral etiology of respiratory papillomatosis, interferon (IFN) following surgical procedures has proved effective [1–10]. Discussion concentrates on the intracellular persistence of viral DNA, following resection of papillomatous lesions, explaining frequent recurrences of these benign tumors [11–15]. This is the intellectual background employing adjuvant therapy with antiviral, antiproliferative and immunomodulating influence [2, 16].

Over the past 4 years we treated 11 patients with recurrent respiratory papillomatosis with interstitial application of IFN in addition to laser-surgical excision using an α-2a-IFN (Roferon®). Six children with an average age of 6.8 years and 5 adults with an average age of 40 years were included in the study. The youngest patient was 10 months old, the oldest 71 years. In all children but one the treatment was primary, whereas all adults had a history of previous treatment. All patients presented with multifocal papillomatous lesions in the pharynx, larynx as well as in the trachea.

The clinical symptoms at therapy onset were more severe in the juvenile type. According to a severity scale proposed by Kashima [7], stage I presents dysphonia only, stage II additionally dyspnea on exertion and stage III dyspnea at rest with stridor and cyanosis. One child was referred after tracheostomy (table 1).

The histology revealed more atypia and dysplasia in adult patients, whilst inflammatory signs were more common in children (table 2).

The average duration of treatment now lies between 24 months for the juvenile group and 31 months for the adult group (table 3). During that time each patient of both groups had 8 laser-surgical operations with or without papilloma detection, thus averaging at 3- to 4-monthly intervals. Every child received 5 applications of IFN, which means more than during every second session. With the adult patients the average number of injections was 2. Apart from influenza-like symptoms no other side effects of intralesional IFN injections were recorded.

Table 1. Patients with laryngotracheal papillomatosis	Papillomatosis laser + IFN injection (Roferon®)	Juvenile (n = 6)	Adult (n = 5)
	Age, years	6.8	40.0
	Previous treatment	1	5
	Clinical degree of symptoms		
	I Dysphonia	–	4
	II Dys-/aphonia Dyspnea	1	1
	III Dyspnea Stridor Cyanosis	5	–
	with tracheostomy	3	

Table 2. Histology at therapy onset	Histology at therapy onset	Juvenile (n = 6)	Adult (n = 5)
	Dyskeratosis	2	3
	Atypia	1	2
	Dysplasia	–	3
	Viral inclusion bodies	3	–
	Round cell infiltrates	4	–

Table 3. Plan of treatment with combined laser surgery and IFN injections	Therapy	Juvenile (n = 6)	Adult (n = 5)
	Duration of treatment, months	24	31
	Operations (CO_2 laser), patients/total	8/45	8/40
	IFN injections (Roferon®), patients/total	5/32	2/8

Table 4. Results of treatment

Results of treatment laser + IFN injection (Roferon®)	Juvenile			Adult		
	n = 6	months	IFN	n = 5	months	IFN
Treatment concluded	1/6	48	1	4/5	46	6
Treatment not concluded	5/6			1/5		
Partial remission	2/5	27	15			
		7	2			
Complete remission	3/5	7	3	1/1	8	2
Recurrence	1/3	10	4			
Again complete remission	1/1	16	3			

The conception consists of laser-surgical resection of the papillomatous lesion followed by interstitial injection of 3 million units of Roferon into the zone of coagulation. In more multifocal papilloma manifestations of the larynx and trachea, a progression in smaller steps at about 6- to 8-weekly intervals is recommended. This reduces the occurrence of adhesions in the anterior commissure and allows higher local concentrations of IFN without exceding the total dose of 3 million units per session.

In all cases adjuvant IFN therapy proved to respond with no initial failure (table 4). In 1 child and 4 adults, the treatment has been concluded after 4 years with no signs of tumor recurrence. Of the remaining patients – 1 adult, 5 children – 2 children suffering from extensive papillomatosis of the upper aerodigestive tract were brought to partial remission with definite control over the disease for 27 months after 11 IFN injections and for 7 months after 2 IFN injections. The remaining adult and 3 children achieved complete remission after therapy onset for 8 and 7 months, respectively. In 1 of these children, however, a recurrence became symptomatic after a complete remission period of 10 months. After recurrent IFN application, it is now tumor-free for 16 months.

In conclusion, the first choice of treatment of recurrent respiratory papillomatosis is laser-surgical excision. Adjuvant interstitial IFN injection presents as an effective beneficial addition, and is virtually without side effects.

References

1 Bomholt A, Oestergaard B, Horn T: Lightmicroscopical features of interferon-alpha-treated laryngeal papillomatosis in adults. Acta Otolaryngol (Stockh) 1986;102:131–135.
2 Crockett DM, McCabe BF, Lusk RP, Mixon JH: Side effects and toxicity of interferon in the treatment of recurrent respiratory papillomatosis. Ann Otol Rhinol Laryngol 1987;96:601–607.
3 Goebel U, Arnold W, Wahn V, Freuner J, Jurgens H, Cantell K: Comparison of human fibroblast and leukocyte interferon in the treatment of severe laryngeal papillomatosis in children. Eur J Pediatr 1981;137:175–176.
4 Goepfert H, Sessions RB, Gutterman JU, Cangir A, Dichtel WJ, Sulek M: Leucocyte interferon in patients with juvenile laryngeal papillomatosis. Ann Otol Rhinol Laryngol 1982;91: 431–436.
5 Haglund S, Lundquist PG, Cantell K, Strander H: Interferon therapy in juvenile laryngeal papillomatosis. Arch Otolaryngol 1981;107:327–332.
6 Healy GB, Gelber RD, Trowbridge AL, Grundfast KM, Ruben R, Price KN: Treatment of recurrent respiratory papillomatosis with human leucocyte interferon. N Engl J Med 1988;319: 401–407.
7 Kashima H, Leventhal B, Dedo H, Gardiner L, McCabe BF, Richardson R, Whisnant J, Clark K, Donovan D, Goepfert H, Mounts P, Singleton G, Wold D, Cohen S, Fearon B, Lusk R, Muntz H, Weck P, Yonkers A: Interferon alpha-N1 (Wellferon)® in juvenile onset recurrent respiratory papillomatosis: Results of a randomized study in twelve collaborative institutions. Laryngoscope 1988;98:334–340.
8 McCabe BF, Clark KF: Interferon and laryngeal papillomatosis. The Iowa experience. Ann Otol Rhinol Laryngol 1983;92:2–7.
9 Schouten TJ, Weimar W, Bos JH, Bos CE, Cremers CWRJ, Schellekens H: Treatment of juvenile laryngeal papillomatosis with two types of interferon. Laryngoscope 1982;92:686–688.
10 Sessions RB, Dichtel WS, Goepfert H: Treatment of recurrent respiratory papillomatosis with interferon. Ear Nose Throat J 1984;63:488–493.
11 Abramson AL, Steinberg BM, Winkler B: Laryngeal papillomatosis: Clinical, histopathologic and molccular studies. Laryngoscope 1987;97:678–685.
12 Boyle WF, Riggs JL, Oshiro LS, Lenette EH: Electron microscopic identification of papova virus in laryngeal papilloma. Laryngoscope 1973;83:1102–1108.
13 Braun L, Kashima H, Eggleston J, Shah K: Demonstration of papillomavirus antigen in paraffin sections of laryngeal papillomas. Laryngoscope 1982;92:640–643.
14 Stremlau A: Humane Papillomviren (HPV) in der HNO-Heilkunde. HNO 1993;41:A15–A20.
15 Terry RM, Lewis FA, Griffiths S, Wells M, Bird CC: Demonstration of human papillomavirus types 6 and 11 in juvenile laryngeal papillomatosis by in-situ DNA hybridization. J Pathol 1987;153:245–248.
16 Isaacs A, Lindenmann J: Virus interference. I. The interferon. Proc R Soc Lond 1957;147: 258–267.

Prof. Dr. C. Herberhold, Universitäts-HNO-Klinik Bonn, Sigmund-Freud-Strasse 25, D–53105 Bonn (Germany)

Rudert H, Werner JA (eds): Lasers in Otorhinolaryngology, and in Head and Neck Surgery.
Adv Otorhinolaryngol. Basel, Karger, 1995, vol 49, pp 170–173

....

Endoscopic Management of Bilateral Recurrent Nerve Paralysis with the CO$_2$ Laser

Tadeus Nawka

Medizinische Fakultät der Humboldt-Universität zu Berlin, Universitätsklinikum
Charité, Universitäts-HNO-Klinik/Abteilung Phoniatrie, Berlin, Deutschland

Bilateral immobilisation of the vocal folds has various reasons. Predominantly, a resection of the thyroid gland in the patients' history will be found as a cause. The nerve injury is most often the reason for paralysis and the inability to open the glottis during respiration. Furthermore, long-term intubation after skull injury is often found etiologically. Other reasons for midline fixation of the vocal folds due to myasthenia, rheumatoid arthritis, gout, mumps, lupus erythematosus disseminatus, or Reiter's disease occur infrequently and may more often lead to ankylosis of the crico-arytenoid joint [1], than to a recurrent nerve paralysis.

A number of methods have been described in the literature about how to operate on bilateral recurrent nerve paralysis since Thornell's [2] report in 1948 about performing it endoscopically. The idea of removing the arytaenoid cartilage proved to be successful throughout the following years [3, 4] and even up to the present.

The 1950s through 1960s were dominated by surgery which took an external approach to the larynx by thyrotomy or lateral access to the arytaenoid. A major disadvantage of these methods is the nearly regularly performed tracheostomy which causes the patient greater morbidity.

Since the advent of the laser two general methods of endoscopic glottal dilation have been established: cordectomy and arytaenoidectomy. In practice, in most of the cases when this operation is performed both methods are combined; the other structure will be included in the resection, respectively. The method of arytaenoidectomy described by Ossoff et al. [5, 6] or Lim [7] appeared to be most promising. The arytaenoid cartilage had been either vaporised or isolated, removed and separated from the vocal fold. The vocal fold itself was trimmed at the resection margin.

Many authors pointed out that the main problem arises from the dilemma between a poor voice and sufficient breathing or vice versa. But there will be no doubt that the maintenance of a good airway is of superior importance. On the other hand, keeping the voice at a good communication level is one of the most desirable goals in the treatment. It is important to provide precise and reproducible information about the results in order to be able to decide on the preferable method. Only a few authors provide functional data of the results [8–11]. In order to consider ventilation, simple but sensitive methods can be applied in the clinical routine. The problem about how to describe the quality of the voice is not yet solved.

Patients and Methods

During the past 6 years, from 1987 through 1993, altogether 74 patients were operated on at the Charité Hospital because of bilateral vocal fold fixation. The reasons were thyroidectomy, multiple thyroidectomies, prolonged intubation after skull and brain damage, or neurologic disorders. Most of the patients were women. At the time of operation the patients' ages ranged from 12 to 80 years. Subjective assessment of the ventilation abilities during exertion and objective findings of pulmonary functions were examined in order to confirm the indication for an operation.

The surgical procedure applied was not equal in all cases but underwent modifications corresponding to the experience acquired. The arytaenoid cartilage is isolated by the laser and excised. The elastic conus of the subglottis and the posterior third of the vocal fold are vaporised. This method, used on approximately the first 20 patients, was then modified. Now, in our operation technique, the caudal part of the vocal fold's mucosa is preserved and sutured to the false vocal fold, thereby covering quite a large part of the open wound. As a rule, a tracheostomy is not performed. Already by the end of the operation, the glottic region is wider than before. A slight edema may occur, which can be controlled by steroids and antibiotics given perioperatively.

The extent of the excision can be adjusted to the requirements of the patient's situation. It is also possible to remove only parts of the arytenoid and the vocal fold or, after resection of the whole cartilage, to simply incise the vocal fold and the conus elasticus without resecting its membranaceous part.

Postoperative hospitalization is necessary for about 7 days in order to control edema and fibrin formation. At times, additional surgical therapy is required. Indirect microsurgical removal of fibrin and granulation polyps under local anesthesia should be a part of the surgeon's operative repertoire.

Results

In a fifth (16) of the cases we had to perform more than one procedure. In the second session, where necessary, the vocal fold of the same side was generally removed or laterally sutured. Contralateral cordectomies or arytenoidectomies should be avoided as long as possible.

Table 1. Results of the respiratory function before and after operation obtained from the data of 74 cases in which laser arytaenoidectomy had been performed

	FEV$_1$/FVC %	Peak flow %
Preoperatively	70.91 ± 20.87	36.50 ± 13.46
Postoperatively	83.97 ± 16.79	56.89 ± 18.88

Means and SD in percent from the normal value for the forced expiratory volume per second in relation to the forced vital capacity (FEV$_1$/FVC) and the peak flow.

All of the 12 patients who were tracheotomised preoperatively were decannulated. In only one case of a malignant struma with bilateral vocal fold fixation after radiation, we failed to prevent a tracheotomy. Thus, in 73 of 74 cases the laser operation was successful. The results of respiratory function are provided in table 1.

To describe the voice function the speaking profiles reflecting the ability of enhancing the intensity have been evaluated. The mean maximal phonation intensity decreases from 73 ± 4.8 to 71 ± 3.8 dB. This small difference is statistically not significant. According to a four point graded (0 through 3) RBH (roughness, breathiness, hoarseness) scale [12] the degree of hoarseness increased from a mean of 1.87 to 2.1.

Discussion

It is obvious that the intralaryngeal approach for restoring the adequacy of the airway after bilateral recurrent nerve palsy is to be favored from the surgical and functional point of view. The operation is limited to the very obturating structures, the arytenoid and the vocal fold. Removal of the whole arytenoid cartilage results finally in a more stable hole for breathing. According to the author's earlier experience the removal of the vocal fold only [13] or incision at the posterior part is less reliable. Laser arytaenoidectomy, together with the posterior vocal fold, is a method that can be adjusted to the needs of the patient, i.e. to the extent of the respiratory restriction.

The procedure of endoscopic intralaryngeal suturing may appear cumbersome, but is very beneficial during the postoperative course. The formation of fibrin or, later, granulation tissue which we observed earlier is now markedly reduced.

The ventilation function is of primary interest in the results, whereas both of the other laryngeal functions, closure during swallowing and phonation, should be maintained as far as possible. The intention to create a better airway without disturbing the voice always leads to the compromise that the one cannot be achieved without affecting the other. It remains a dilemma. Hence, respiration receives preference. Otherwise, the indication to the operative procedure of arytaenoidectomy should not be stipulated. It is important to know how far the airway compromise can be reduced. The improvement of the peak flow of about 20% in comparison to the preoperative findings has been proven by regression analysis. 57% from the normal peak flow as a mean result seems to be a reasonable measure which most properly reflects the actual situation. After widening the glottis by lateralisations of one vocal fold, it can reach a maximum of about half its normal area.

References

1　Gerhardt HJ: Zur Remobilisierung einer Ankylose im Krikoarytaenoidgelenk. HNO Praxis 1982;7:249–255.
2　Thornell WC: Intralaryngeal approach for arytenoidectomy in bilateral abductor vocal cord paralysis. Arch Otolaryngol 1948;47:505–8.
3　Whicker JH, Devine KD: Long-term results of Thornell arytenoidectomy in the surgical treatment of bilateral vocal cord paralysis. Laryngoscope 1972;82:1331–1336.
4　Kleinsasser O: Mikrolaryngoskopie und endolaryngeale Mikrochirurgie: Technik und typische Befunde. 3., völlig neu überarb Aufl. Stuttgart, Schattauer, 1991.
5　Ossoff RH, Sisson GA, Duncavage JA, Moselle HI, Andrews PE, McMillan WG: Endoscopic laser arytaenoidectomy for the treatment of bilateral vocal cord paralysis. Laryngoscope 1984;94:1293–1297.
6　Ossoff RH, Duncavage JA, Shapshay SM, Krespi YP, Sisson GA Sr: Endoscopic laser arytenoidectomy revisited. Ann Otol Rhinol Laryngol 1990;99:764–71.
7　Lim RY: Laser Arytenoidectomy. Arch Otolaryngol 1985;111:262–263.
8　Dennis DP, Kashima H: Carbon dioxide laser posterior cordectomy for treatment of bilateral vocal cord paralysis. Ann Otol Rhinol Laryngol 1989;98:930–934.
9　Fischer S, Wendler J, Anders L, Walch I, Seidner W, Rauhut A, Schuchardt P: Funktionelle Befunde nach glottiserweiternden Operationen. Wiss Z Humboldt Universität zu Berlin, Math.-Nat. R. XXXIII 1984;2/3:168–171.
10　Geterud Å, Ejnell H, Stenborg R, Bake B: Long-term results with a simple surgical treatment of bilateral vocal cord paralysis. Laryngoscope 1990;100:1005–1008.
11　Stange G, Holm C, Schumann K: Funktionelle Resultate endolaryngealer Lateralfixationen. Laryngol Rhinol 1974;53:943–949.
12　Nawka T, Anders LC, Wendler J: Die auditive Beurteilung heiserer Stimmen nach dem RBH-System. Sprache Stimme Gehör, 1994;3:130–133.
13　Eckel HE: Die laserchirurgische mikrolaryngoskopische Glottiserweiterung zur Behandlung der beidseitigen Rekurrensparese. Laryngorhinootologie 1991;70:17–20.

Priv.-Doz. Dr. med. Tadeus Nawka, Medizinische Fakultät der Humboldt-Universität zu Berlin, Universitätsklinikum Charité, Universitäts-HNO-Klinik/Abteilung Phoniatrie, D–10098 Berlin (Germany)

Rudert H, Werner JA (eds): Lasers in Otorhinolaryngology, and in Head and Neck Surgery.
Adv Otorhinolaryngol. Basel, Karger, 1995, vol 49, pp 174–175

....

Posterior Cordotomy by CO$_2$ Laser Surgery for Bilateral Vocal Cord Paralysis: Kashima's Technique and Modified Technique

C. Herberhold, P. Hück

Universitätsklinik für Hals-, Nasen- und Ohrenkranke der Universität Bonn,
Deutschland

Microlaryngoscopic posterior cordotomy by CO$_2$ laser surgery as a treatment for bilateral vocal cord paralysis has first been described by Dennis and Kashima [1] in 1989. The vocal cord is cut off the vocal process of the arytaenoid cartilage and shortens spontaneously leaving space in the area of the posterior commissure. Thus, it provides here a wider airway without worsening voice quality by providing contact of the vocal folds in their anterior parts.

Up to September 1991, we were dealing with bilateral vocal cord paralysis by doing a craniolateral fixation of the vocal cord microlaryngoscopically [2]. This procedure provides good results in respiratory function and voice but is difficult and intensive in time. Since we had been using endoscopic laser surgery and fibrin glue for fixing the mucosa, it had become somewhat easier. Later we shifted to the Kashima technique.

Since we learned in our patients that the initially good results disappear in some cases by rescarring of the incision, which makes it hard to recognize the former place of the cordotomy, we modified Kashima's technique keeping his principles:

We cut off the vocal cord unilaterally not only transversely from the vocal process of the arytaenoid cartilage but mobilized it additionally from the thyroid cartilage in about a third of its length. Thus, the vocal cord can retract by a greater distance leaving more place for respiration in the dorsal commissure. The other advantage is that in the process of healing it doesn't have contact with its former bed and is thus not pulled back by rescarring.

In 25 treated patients aged between 3 and 89 years, we have used the modified technique 22 times. Tracheotomy was not required in any of our patients. In 19 patients the airway resistance could be measured by spirometry. Voice function and degree of dyspnea were assessed subjectively by the patient, by measurement of the tone and dynamic range of voice and by respiration tests.

In those patients who had undergone the modified procedure, 18% didn't show a measurable improvement of respiratory function, 18% had little improvement up to 10% and 64% had a FEV_1 postoperatively which reached from 110 to 204% (median 115%) of the preoperative figure. The subjective parameter of feeling dyspnea under physical stress improved in all patients.

Voice quality worsened in only 1 patient, there was no change in 2 patients. Surprisingly, there was an improvement of voice in 10 patients. This may be due to the increased vital capacity (median 2.43 before and 2.63 liters after treatment) which allows louder and longer speech.

Conclusion

Treatment of bilateral vocal cord paralysis has to put emphasizis on the respiratory function and preservation of voice quality. According to our experience, modified technique of CO_2 laser cordotomy freeing the vocal cord not only from the vocal process of the arytaenoid cartilage but also partially from the thyroid cartilage improves the measurable respiratory function as well as the subjective degree of dyspnea and voice quality.

References

1   Dennis DP, Kashima H: Carbon dioxide laser posterior cordectomy for treatment of bilateral vocal cord paralysis. Ann Otol Rhinol Laryngol 1989;98:930–934.
2   Langnickel R, Coburg E: Die endolaryngeale Lateralfixation des Stimmbandes zur Behandlung der beiderseitigen Posticusparese. HNO 1970;8:239–242.

Prof. Dr. C. Herberhold, Universitäts-HNO-Klinik Bonn, Sigmund-Freud-Strasse 25, D–53105 Bonn (Germany)

Rudert H, Werner JA (eds): Lasers in Otorhinolaryngology, and in Head and Neck Surgery.
Adv Otorhinolaryngol. Basel, Karger, 1995, vol 49, pp 176–178

....

Laser Surgical Techniques for the Treatment of Glottic Stenoses

Heinrich Rudert

Department of Otorhinolaryngology, Head and Neck Surgery,
University of Kiel, Germany

Operative procedures for the treatment of glottic stenoses belong to the large chapter of surgery of stenoses which was intentionally not systematically discussed during this meeting because the laser is only useful for the treatment of soft tissue stenoses caused by scars. Stenoses of the cartilaginous skeleton of the larynx and the trachea cannot be treated with the laser. Circular scar tissue stenosis is best treated by star-shaped incisions. This way intact mucosa remains to reepithelize the surface of the cut which in turn prevents restenosis.

The most common and important soft tissue stenosis is *bilateral paralysis of the recurrent nerve*. This article is the result of a 25-years experience with different methods and is intended to supplement the operative methods for glottic widening [1].

The high number of external and endolaryngeal operative procedures reflects the unsatisfying therapeutic situation when dealing with bilateral recurrent nerve paralysis. Present operations with an external approach are a variation of the technique initially described by King [2] and Woodman [3]. They yield different results and are often only successful in the hands of their authors. When I came to Cologne in 1969 as a senior resident, Kleinsasser [4] had just developed his modification of Thornell's endolaryngeal arytenoidectomy with a reliable outcome. I also used this technique and continued until 1976 in Kiel with equally good results. The CO_2 laser has been used instead of cold cutting instruments since the 1980s. Its advantages are the superior hemostasis and the reduced edema especially when using modern micromanipulators with a focus diameter of 0.25 mm. For safety reasons all patients undergo tracheostomy beforehand as recommended by Kleinsasser [5]. The tracheostoma is closed after a few days.

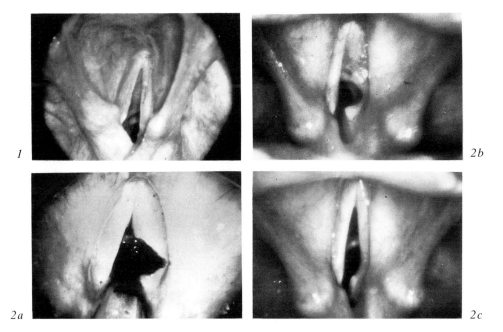

1

2a

2b

2c

Fig. 1. Glottis 8 months after arytenoidectomy.

Fig. 2. a Glottis immediately after posterior chordectomy as described by Dennis and Kashima [7]. The result is a large triangular opening in the dorsal glottic area. *b* Glottis 6 days after posterior chordectomy. *c* Glottis 6 months after posterior chordectomy. The scaring process changed the glottis to a one-sided oval-shaped hole.

We follow the technique as described by Kleinsasser [5] but using the CO_2 laser. First, a triangular field of the arytenoid covering mucosa is excised. Then, we completely extirpate the arytenoid cartilage. With the CO_2 laser, the muscular layer is separated directly at the cartilage without major bleeding. If necessary, one can then remove parts of the thyreoarytaenoid muscle submucosally. The conus elasticus is incised caudally in the dorsal third of the vocal cord. The vocal cord is thereby mobilized. It is fixated by two or three stitches to the cranial cutting edge of the initially resected triangular piece of mucosa. We do not vaporize the arytenoid as Ossoff et al. [6] recommend since high temperatures are generated with this method which cause thermal damage of the neighboring tissue.

Since 2 years, we have also tried a different method described by Dennis and Kashima [7] as posterior chordectomy. It is a simple and therefore attractive procedure. A CO_2 laser incision is directed from the processus muscularis laterally. A triangular piece of tissue is removed with the base towards the free vocal cord margin and the tip laterally in the muscle. This results in a large triangular opening in the dorsal glottic area which shrinks after a few weeks. The scaring process changes the glottis to a one-sided oval-shaped hole. It is not always sufficient for respiration so that in some cases the contralateral side has to be treated or the removal of the arytenoid has to be considered (fig. 1, 2). It has to be shown if the additional vertical incision from the tip of the resected triangle anteriorly results in a larger opening as recently described by Nawka [1].

Conclusion

For arytenoidectomy as described by Kleinsasser [4], the use of a CO_2 laser is the safest method to treat bilateral recurrent nerve paralysis. According to Dennis and Kashima [7] posterior chordectomy is suitable mainly for minor and almost compensated glottic stenoses where an only slight enlargement of the glottis is necessary. Other indications are recurrent nerve paralysis in patients with incurable mediastinal or pulmonal malignancies and an anticipated short survival. In these cases, a tracheostomy can be avoided. The advantage of the posterior chordectomy is a short operating time of only a few minutes so that it is less stressful for the patients than complete arytenoidectomy.

References

1   Nawka T: Endoscopic management of bilateral recurrent nerve paralysis with the CO_2 laser. Adv Otorhinolaryngol. Basel, Karger, 1995, vol 49, pp 170–173.
2   King BT: A new and function revtoring operation for bilateral abductor cord paralysis. JAMA 1939;112:814–823.
3   Woodman D: A modification of the extralaryngeal approach to arytenoidectomy for bilateral abductor paralysis. Arch Otolaryngol 1946;43:63–65.
4   Kleinsasser O: Endolaryngeale Arytaenoidektomie und submuköse Hemichordektomie zur Erweiterung der Glottis bei bilateraler Abductorparese. Monatsschr Ohrenheilkd 1986;102: 443–446.
5   Kleinsasser O, Nolte E: Endolaryngeale Arytaenoidektomie und submuköse partielle Chordektomie bei bilateralen Stimmlippenlähmungen (Bericht über 120 Fälle). Laryngol Rhinol Otol 1981;60:397–401.
6   Ossoff RH, Sisson GA, Duncavage JA, Moselle HI, Andreus PE, McMillan WG: Endoscopic laser arytenoidectomy for the treatment of bilateral vocal cord paralysis. Laryngoscope 1984; 94:1293–1297.
7   Dennis DP, Kashima H: Carbon dioxide laser posterior cordectomy for treatment of bilateral vocal cord paralysis. Ann Otol Rhinol Laryngol 1989;98:930–934.

Prof. Dr. Heinrich Rudert, Department of Otorhinolaryngology, Head and Neck Surgery, University of Kiel, Arnold-Heller-Strasse 14, D–24105 Kiel (Germany)

Rudert H, Werner JA (eds): Lasers in Otorhinolaryngology, and in Head and Neck Surgery.
Adv Otorhinolaryngol. Basel, Karger, 1995, vol 49, pp 179–181

....

Treatment of a Tracheal Stenosis with a CO₂ Laser Using a Rigid ArthroLase™ CO₂ Wave Guide System

A Case Report

H. Schmidt [a], *K. Hörmann* [b], *N. Stasche* [a], *U. Reineke* [b]

[a] ENT Department (Head: Dr. *N. Stasche*), Klinikum Kaiserslautern, and
[b] University ENT Department Mannheim (Head: Prof. *K. Hörmann*), Germany

For endotracheal splinting in cases of tracheal stenosis T-like Montgomery stents are reliable. A possible complication is developing cranial and caudal granulations.

Generally, the removal of the granulations by laser surgery is not difficult. Nevertheless, the following case history illustrates that under special circumstances problems may arise.

Case History

In 1973, we presented a 52-year-old patient with polytrauma and long-term artificial respiration. Several tracheoplasties due to a long tracheal stenosis followed.

In 1989, an emergency tracheotomy was necessary due to a strong tracheomalacy. Subsequently, a gradual bougination starting at the cricoid, ending 2 cm above the bifurcation of the trachea with an extended Montgomery T tubus was done. We achieved a tracheal lumen of 16 Charrière (diameter = 5.33 mm). After this therapy, the patient was free of dyspnea with a normal voice.

In 1993, the patient came with inspiratory and expiratory stridor under emergency circumstances caused by an infection of the upper respiratory tract.

We diagnosed a strictly subglottically positioned constricting granulation which obliterated the cranial end of the tracheal cannula.

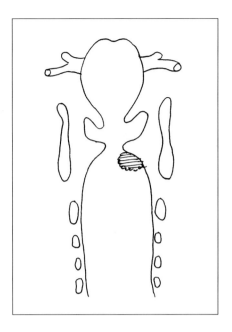

Fig. 1. The subglottically located granulation in the larynx in a vertical section.

Results

The removal of the granulation under conventional proceedings including microlaryngoscopy and CO_2 laser microscopic transmission failed. Figure 1 shows the granulation in the larynx in a vertical section. It demonstrates that a complete removal of this tissue would include the resection of a functioning vocal cord using microlaryngoscopic approach. We decided to resect the granulation using the ArthroLase™ CO_2 wave guide system. This equipment is common in arthroscopic surgery. This system represents a hollow probe containing an optical wave guide composed of special ceramics and a metal coating. During operation, the probe is fixed in an outer metal cover permitting permanent rinsing with gaseous CO_2. The tip of the probe allows a straight and a rectangular radiation. The length is 120 mm. Through a special plug device, it can easily be connected to a CO_2 laser system. With this equipment, it was possible to remove the obliterating granulation using local anesthesia under visual control using a 70° Hopkins endoscope.

During the operation, we had an output power of 20 W in the continuous-wave status. Arising smoke was exhausted through a transnasal catheter. The entire operation lasted 15 min.

Follow-up investigations didn't show any recurrence of the described granulations.

Discussion

Using the rectangular probe of the ArthroLase™ CO_2 wave guide system, removal of the subglottically located granulations was possible without damaging the vocal cords.

The rectangular transmission system permits easily to reach all important regions of the trachea and the larynx in patients with tracheotomy. Regions which were previously difficult to reach can now certainly be inspected using the described system. We can operate under local anesthesia, and use under outpatient conditions is possible.

The power decrease when using the rectangular transmission system is minimal.

A major disadvantage is the scattering of shredded tissue and fluids on the tip of the probe. This leads to divergence and absorption of the laser beam resulting in a power decrease and heating of the probe tip.

Contact with the surrounding tissue might occur due to the free-hand handling of the transmission system. The consequences are additional carbonization and further loss of power.

Extensive operations of restless patients require more than one of the single-use transmission systems.

We treated 3 patients with tracheal granulations. We consider the Arthro-Lase™ wave guide system an elegant alternative to the traditional CO_2 laser system for removing granulations of the trachea in patients after tracheotomy.

Dr. H. Schmidt, HNO-Klinik, Klinikum Kaiserslautern, Friedrich-Engels-Strasse 25, D–67653 Kaiserslautern (Germany)

Rudert H, Werner JA (eds): Lasers in Otorhinolaryngology, and in Head and Neck Surgery.
Adv Otorhinolaryngol. Basel, Karger, 1995, vol 49, pp 182–184

....

Laser Arytenoidectomy in the Treatment of Bilateral Vocal Cord Paralysis

Zygmunt Szmeja, Jerzy G. Wójtowicz

ENT Clinic, Medical Academy, Poznań, Poland

The introduction of surgical laser into larynx microsurgery [1–3, 7, 8] has made the resection of the posterior vocal cord together with the arytenoid cartilage possible. This method allows one to carry out a fast and practically bloodless operation with minimal postoperative edema of the surrounding tissues.

It should be emphasized that in the preoperative period, tracheotomy, as the stage preceding the surgery, was not performed as lack of edema of the operation field allowed this surgery to be performed by the intralaryngeal method [4–7] without any problems of breathing disturbances.

Material and Method

Since November 1990, at the Clinic of Otolaryngology of the Medical Academy in Poznań, 30 arytenoidectomies (18 on the right side, 12 on the left side) were performed by means of a CO_2 laser in patients with bilateral paralysis of the vocal cords. In this group there were 22 women (in 1 case the operation was performed twice – excision of the right arytenoid cartilage, and in the second the left arytenoid cartilage) (76.7%) and 7 men (23.3%), age range 28–71 years, mean age 46.7 ± 13.5 years (44.8 ± 15.5 for women and 50.0 ± 9.5 for men). Three patients underwent tracheotomy before being admitted to the Clinic.

In the etiology of vocal cord paralysis there are complications arising from surgical treatment of the thyroid gland (26 cases dominated, with some years of medical history, in 1 case medical history of 20 years, 2 posttraumatic cases, 1 case of bilateral glomus caroticum tumor).

The operation was performed under general intratracheal anesthesia with the use of a Laser-Flex-Mt tube (Mallinckrodt Company). Microsurgery of the larynx was performed using a typical modo Kleinsasser set with the help of a Weerdy surgical laryngoscope (Storz Company). Arytenoidectomy was performed using an OP-Mi 11 surgical microscope (Opton Company) with a focal lens of 400 mm, connected to a micromanipulator. This micromanipulator allows a concentrated and scattered laser beam compatible to the focus of the lens of surgical microscope to be received. A difocused laser beam of 10 W and a spot diameter within $\varnothing = 2-5$ mm was used.

While making incisions on soft tissues with the laser beam, a concentrated 10-watt beam was used in interrupted mode with a single impulse time of 0.1 s or an uninterrupted work mode.

During the operation, the arytenoid cartilage was excised together with 1/3 of the posterior part of the operated vocal cord.

Results

In all patients postoperative recovery was correct and breathing difficulties were not observed after extubation. In the postoperative period, antibiotic treatment was used and corticosteroid preparations were administered orally over a period of 2–3 days. Laryngoscopic control examinations were performed a day after the operation and a wide lumen of air through the operative field was observed. Bleeding in the postoperative period did not occur, we did not observe choking. After 2–10 days' hospital stay, the patients were released in good condition and those with previously performed tracheotomy were decannulated. After treatment wide air lumen through the glottis was observed in all the cases. Patients are under the care of the Laryngological Polyclinic. At the control examination, narrowing of the lumen of the larynx was not observed, and the laryngological picture presented the process of healing of the operation area without granulation.

Conclusions

Laser arytenoidectomy allows good results of the breathing and phonation function. No changes of granulation proliferation were observed at the size of the CO_2 laser treatment.

Lack of reaction to laser section allows operations to be performed by means of endoscopy in patients who did not undergo a tracheotomy.

References

1 Eskew JR, Bailey BJ: Laser arytenoidectomy for bilateral vocal cord paralysis. Otolaryngol Head Neck Surg 1983;91:294.
2 Katin LI, Tucker JA: Laser supraarytenoidectomy for laryngomalacia with apnea. Trans Pa Acad Ophtalmol Otolaryngol 1990;42:985.
3 Lim RY: Laser arytenoidectomy. Arch Otolaryngol 1985;111:262.
4 Ossoff RH, Duncavage JA, Shapsky SM, Krespi YP, Sisson GA Sr: Endoscopic laser arytenoidectomy revisited. Ann Otol Rhinol Laryngol 1990;99:764.
5 Ossoff RH, Karlan MS, Sisson GA: Endoscopic laser arytenoidectomy. Laser Surg Med 1983;2:293.
6 Ossoff RH, Sisson GA, Duncavage JA, Moselle HI, Andrews PE, McMillan WG: Endoscopic laser arytenoidectomy for the treatment of bilateral vocal cord paralysis. Laryngoscope. 1984;94:1293.
7 Prasad U: CO_2 surgical laser in the management of bilateral vocal cord paralysis. J Laryngol Otol 1985;99:891.
8 Tate LP, Newman HC, Cullen JM, Sweeney C: Neodymium (Nd):YAG laser surgery in the equine larynx: A pilot study. Lasers Surg Med 1986;6:473.

Zygmunt Szmeja, MD, ENT-Clinic, Medical Academy, ul. Przybyszewskiego 49,
PL–60–355 Poznań (Poland)

Rudert H, Werner JA (eds): Lasers in Otorhinolaryngology, and in Head and Neck Surgery.
Adv Otorhinolaryngol. Basel, Karger, 1995, vol 49, pp 185–190

....

Transoral Laser Surgery for Oral Carcinoma

Hans Edmund Eckel[a], *Peter Volling*[a], *Olaf Ebeling*[a], *Ima Schneider*[a],
Walter Franz Thumfart[b]

[a] Department of Oto-Rhino-Laryngology, University of Cologne, Germany;
[b] Department of Oto-Rhino-Laryngology, University of Innsbruck, Austria

In recent years, transoral resections of the oral cavity and oropharyngeal malignancies have gained new importance by the introduction of the CO_2 surgical laser [1–7]. It provides advantages relating to its hemostatic effects and precision of tissue ablation [8, 9] and has therefore led to a renaissance of transoral surgery. Functional results following transoral laser surgery have been reported to be excellent [4, 7]. The surgical concept for the treatment of infiltrating oral cavity and oropharynx carcinoma used at the Department of Otorhinolaryngology, University of Cologne, Germany, is transoral resection of the tumor and discontinuous, asynchronous neck dissection. This study investigated the results of transoral laser surgery and discontinuous, asynchronous neck dissection in a series of 117 patients.

Patients and Methods

One hundred and seventeen patients with infiltrating oral carcinoma were treated for cure with transoral resection of the primary and staged neck dissection. Patients with carcinoma in situ and superficial carcinoma not at risk to spread to the regional lymph nodes were not included in this study. Twenty-eight patients were female and 89 were male. Mean age of all patients was 56 years, range 28–85 years. All patients were followed up for 3–7 years from the onset of tumor-directed therapy.

Prior to any decision on the adequate treatment of their tumors, all patients underwent panendoscopy of the upper aerodigestive tract to allow detailed and exact assessment of the tumor and to rule out secondary coexisting primaries. All patients with histologically proven squamous cell carcinoma of the oral cavity and oropharynx presenting at our institution were submitted to transoral laser resection of the primary if the following conditions were met: (1) Sufficient general health condition of the patient to allow surgery under general anesthesia. (2) Adequate tumor exposure. (3) Absence of bone invasion as judged from the clinical aspect, conventional X-rays or computed tomography scans. Invasion of the periosteum without infiltration of the mandibula, however, was not considered to be an indication for extraoral surgery. (4) Absence of deep invasion of the primary into the cervical viscera with suspected infiltration of major cervical blood vessels (especially for carcinoma of the tonsils). (5) Resectability of clinically obvious cervical metastases. If lymph node metastases were judged to be unresectable, no surgical treatment of the primary tumor was performed even if the primary seemed amenable to surgical treatment.

All of the transoral interventions were performed under general anesthesia. We used a Heraeus LS 500 CO_2 laser coupled with a Zeiss operating microscope with a 300-mm lens.

Elective treatment of the N0 neck included limited selective or functional neck dissections, while radical neck dissections were only performed for advanced nodal disease with fixation to the surrounding tissues. If the site of the primary suggested the risk of bilateral spread, e.g. in cancers of the tongue or the floor of mouth, simultaneous bilateral neck dissections were performed. Neck dissections were usually performed 1–3 weeks after the resection of the primary. Neck dissections were staged to minimize the risk of fistula formation and to allow for tumor cells in lymphatic capillaries to migrate to the regional lymph nodes prior to their removal. Postoperative radiotherapy was administered in all patients with stage III–IV disease.

Functional Evaluation after Treatment

Thirty-one randomly chosen patients were re-evaluated 6 months after completion of their initial treatment to identify functional impairment resulting from the therapy. The evaluation was conducted using a modified version of Teichgräber's [10] test series for the functional evaluation of oral cavity cancer, adopted for the German language. In a special evaluation form, the actual weight of the patient, continuing pain, activities at home and at work, xerostomia, visible mutilation, disorders of tongue mobility and sensitivity, speech impairment, swallowing disorders and psychological problems were assessed. The documentation was completed by application of a score system that allows for a reliable determination of functional results after treatment of oral cavity carcinoma [11].

Results

Postoperative Healing Process

None of the patients in this series had a tracheostomy as swelling of the adjacent tissues is minimal and the pharyngeal airway is not compromised. Complete reepithelialization of the nonclosed surgical defects was usually complete within 3–6 weeks after transoral surgery, depending largely on the size of the surgical defect. No cases of radiation-induced osteonecrosis of the mandible or of deep neck infections had to be observed in this series.

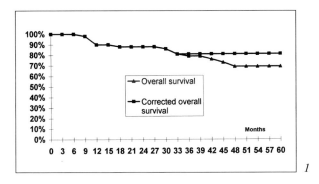

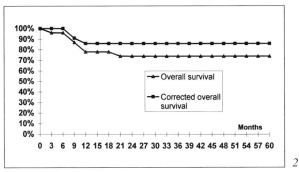

Fig. 1. Survival in patients with stage I and II carcinomas of the oral cavity (n = 42).
Fig. 2. Survival in patients with stage I and II carcinomas of the oropharynx (n = 23).

Complications

Three patients required operative suture ligation of a bleeding vessel during the postoperative period. All had previously had resections of T2/T3 tumors of the oropharynx. These hemorrhages occurred on the third, fifth and sixth postoperative days, respectively. Two patients developed severe trismus following laser resection of carcinoma of the buccal cavity. As both later presented with local recurrences, it remains unclear whether this complication was due to scarry contraction of the cheek or rather an early sign of recurrent disease.

Survival

All patients were followed up for 3 years or more unless they died. Figures 1–4 demonstrate the calculated overall and corrected survival curves according to stage of disease and primary site after 5 years for patients in stages I–III. Tumor-related survival after 5 years is 81% for stage I and II disease of the oral cavity, 86% for stage I and II disease of the oropharynx,

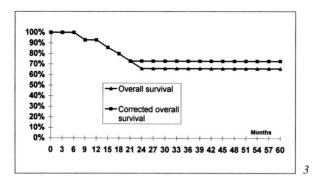

3

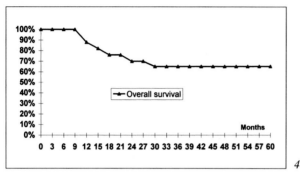

4

Fig. 3. Survival in patients with stage III carcinomas of the oral cavity (n = 15).
Fig. 4. Survival in patients with stage III carcinomas of the oropharynx (n = 17).

73% for stage III disease of the oral cavity, 65% for stage III disease of the oropharynx, and 21% for stage IV disease of the oral cavity and the oropharynx.

Functional Results

Of 31 patients submitted to re-evaluation 6 months after treatment, 16 gained a score in the range of 76–100 (maximum score indicating ideal result = 100). Ten patients reached a score in the range of 51–75 and only 5 patients had a score of 50 or worse. These findings indicate excellent functional results in the majority of our patients and fair results in a minority. Functional outcome depended largely on the site and size of the primary.

Discussion

In contrast to most of the hitherto published studies, our concept for the treatment of cervical nodes in oral carcinoma was curative neck dissection if cervical metastases were clinically obvious and prophylactic neck dissection in the clinically negative neck. The concept of transoral tumor resection and staged discontinuous neck dissection with additional radiotherapy in advanced stages is not a new one [12, 13], but has recently gained strong support by the work and clinical experience of Steiner and co-workers [6, 7]. The advantages of this concept are the following:

(1) No reconstruction of the oral or pharyngeal defect is required. The wound epithelializes from the margins of the defect by second intention. The result is frequently a surgical defect covered by normal oral/pharyngeal mucosa that has functional advantages over transplanted full-thickness skin grafts. This leads to less mobility impairment of the tongue, soft palate or lateral pharyngeal wall than submucous scars following primary wound closure [11]. It is noteworthy that surgical defects resulting from transoral laser resection of the oral carcinoma are very similar, although frequently more extended, to those after simple tonsillectomy in adults. These defects are well known to heal by secondary intention with excellent functional results, and the same applies to intraoral or pharyngeal wounds after transoral laser resection.

(2) Two minor surgical interventions (transoral laser resection of primary and staged neck dissection) replace one major procedure and perioperative mortality is low (no patient in this series died related to tumor-directed treatment). Bleeding during these interventions is usually minimal and transfusions of blood are not required as a rule. Fistula formation does not occur. Tracheostomy is not needed in combination with transoral resection of carcinoma of the oral cavity or oropharynx due to minimal swelling of anatomical structures surrounding the surgical defect. Patients can usually resume their normal diet within 1 or 2 days from surgery.

Specific disadvantages of this concept are the need to perform two surgical interventions (including the need to perform repeated general anesthesia) and prolonged wound healing after resection of extended primaries. Prolonged secondary wound healing, although frequently not painful or otherwise disturbing to the patient, includes the risk of delaying the onset of postoperative radiotherapy.

Conclusion

The combination of microscopically controlled CO_2 laser resection and staged neck dissection offers cure rates comparable to those after radical extraoral surgery. These two minor surgical interventions cause less morbidity than commando-type surgery and lead to low perioperative mortality and morbidity and excellent functional results. Careful patient selection is crucial. Tumors infiltrating the mandible or deeply invading the cervical viscera should be resected via an extraoral approach.

References

1 Schuller DE: Use of the laser in the oral cavity. Otolaryngol Clin North Am 1990;23:31–42.
2 Strong MS, Vaughan CW, Healy GB, Shapshay SM, Jako GJ: Transoral management of localized carcinoma of the oral cavity using the CO_2 laser. Laryngoscope 1979;89:897–905.
3 Carruth JAS: Resection of the tongue with the carbon dioxide laser. J Laryngol Otol 1982;96: 529–543.
4 Panje WR, Scher N, Karnell M: Transoral carbon dioxide laser ablation for cancer, tumors, and other diseases. Arch Otolaryngol Head Neck Surg 1989;115:681–688.
5 Rhys Williams S, Carruth JAS: The role of the carbon dioxide laser in treatment of carcinoma of the tongue. J Laryngol Otol 1988;102:1122–1123.
6 Steiner W, Aurbach G, Ambrosch P: Minimally invasive therapy in otorhinolaryngology and head and neck surgery. Minim Invas Ther 1991;1:57–70.
7 Steiner W: Experience in endoscopic laser surgery of malignant tumours of the upper aerodigestive tract. Adv Otorhinolaryngol. Basel, Karger, 1988, vol 39, pp 135–144.
8 Chu FWK, Silverman S, Dedo HH: CO_2 laser treatment of oral leukoplakia. Laryngoscope 1988;98:125–130.
9 Guerry TL, Silverman S, Dedo HH: Carbon dioxide laser resection of superficial oral carcinoma: Indications, technique, and results. Ann Otol Rhinol Laryngol 1986;95:547–555.
10 Teichgräber J, Bowman J, Goepfert H: New test series for the functional evaluation of oral cavity cancer. Head Neck Surg 1985;8:9–20.
11 Eckel HE, Pitten F, Volling P: Ein Untersuchungsgang zur Beurteilung funktioneller Endzustände nach Behandlung von Karzinomen der Mundhöhle. Laryngol Rhinol Otol 1991;70: 546–551.
12 Leemans CR, Tiwari R, Nauta JJP, Snow GB: Discontinuous vs. incontinuity neck dissection in carcinoma of the oral cavity. Arch Otolaryngol Head Neck Surg 1991;117:1003–1006.
13 Spiro RH, Strong EW: Discontinuous partial glossectomy and radical neck dissection in selected patients with epidermoid carcinoma of the mobile tongue. Am J Surg 1973;126:544–546.

Dr. H.E. Eckel, Universitäts-Hals-Nasen-Ohrenklinik, Joseph-Stelzmann-Strasse 9,
D–50937 Köln (Germany)

Rudert H, Werner JA (eds): Lasers in Otorhinolaryngology, and in Head and Neck Surgery.
Adv Otorhinolaryngol. Basel, Karger, 1995, vol 49, pp 191–195

....

Enoral/Transoral Surgery of Malignancies of the Oral Cavity and the Oropharynx[1]

H. Iro, F. Waldfahrer, K. Gewalt, J. Zenk, A. Altendorf-Hofmann

Department of Oto-Rhino-Laryngology, Head and Neck Surgery
(Head: Prof. *M.E. Wigand*), University of Erlangen-Nuremberg, Germany

Since the end of the last century surgical treatment of malignomas of the oral cavity and the oropharynx has emphasized radical en bloc (segmental) tumor resections. The primary tumor has been removed in continuity with a radical neck dissection. The results of these so-called comando operations, advocated mainly by Martin and Sugarbaker [1] and Conley and von Fränkel [2] can, however, be described as dissappointing referring also to the quality of life of the patients afterwards. During the last 15 years enoral and transoral resections of malignomas of the oral cavity and the oropharynx were increasingly favored.

This technique prefers the physiological preformed route to the transcervical approach through the soft tissues of the neck. Necessary neck dissections are performed either in the same operation discontinuously or in a second step 2 or 3 weeks later, depending on the size and location of the primary tumor.

Since the end of the 1970s, the enoral/transoral techniques of tumor resections in the upper aerodigestive tract together with discontinuously performed functional neck dissections have been carried out in the ENT Department of the University of Erlangen-Nuremberg. In a retrospective study, the results of this tumor management will be demonstrated.

[1] This work was supported by the Johannes and Frieda Marohn Foundation and the Sophie Wallner Foundation, Friedrich Alexander Universität, Erlangen-Nürnberg.

Patients and Methods

In our study the history of 205 patients with squamous cell carcinoma of the oropharynx and 186 patients with squamous cell carcinomas of the oral cavity were analyzed. In the cases of the oropharynx carcinomas 47 patients suffered from stage I or II tumors, 55 from stage III tumors and 103 patients from stage IV tumors [3]. Seventy-nine patients with carcinomas of the oral cavity had stage I or II tumors, 67 patients stage III and 40 patients stage IV tumors.

Treatment
In all patients the primary tumor has been removed by enoral/transoral resection – partly by electrosurgery and partly by applying microscope-coupled CO_2 laser. Depending on the size and the location of the primary tumor, functional neck dissection has been performed either in the same operation discontinuously or in a second step 2 or 3 weeks later.

In stage III and IV, a postoperative percutaneous radiotherapy has been carried out.

Evaluation
The histories of the patients who were operated until 31.12.1990 were retrospectively analyzed passing an especially developed questionnaire. The follow-up period was at least 3 years.

Results

The noncorrected 5-year survival rates of oral cavity carcinomas in tumor stages I and II were 66%, whereas it was 51% in tumor stage II and 34% in stage IV (fig. 1). In the cases of oropharynx carcinomas we reached noncorrected 5-year survival rates of 58% in tumor stages I and II, 41% in stage III and 35% in stage IV with enoral/transoral tumor management (fig. 2).

Discussion

Within the last 15 years, various research groups have published reports on transoral resections which were performed in cases of advanced malignancies in regions of the oral cavity and oropharynx – partly by electrosurgery and partly by applying microscope-coupled CO_2 lasers [4–9]. The oncological results reported are comparable to those achieved by bloc resections and reconstruction of defects by pedicled or microvasculary anastomosed flaps [10–12]. Panje et al. [7] and Steiner [13], in particular, have emphasized the substantially lower degree of impairment of the patient caused by transoral resections, thus rendering unnecessary measures to reconstruct defects. By spontaneous epithelialization of the operated sites, extensive functional maintenance can be

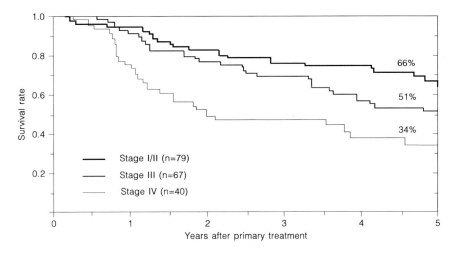

Fig. 1. Survival rate after enoral surgery of malignancies of the oral cavity, combined with neck dissection and postoperative radiotherapy (in cases of stage III and IV). n = 186.

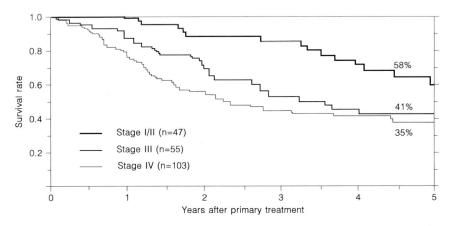

Fig. 2. Survival rate after enoral/transoral surgery of malignancies of the oropharynx, combined with neck dissection and postoperative radiotherapy (in cases of stage III and IV). n = 205.

achieved, with little cosmetic impairment [7]. Strong [9] recommends minimally invasive, conservative transoral resections of carcinomas whenever such an approach is manageable. If tumor margins cannot, however, be clearly outlined or if tumor has penetrated into adjacent soft tissue of the neck, Strong [9] believes that transoral resections are no longer possible. Denecke [14], on the other hand, considers a transoral approach to be essentially feasible, even if the mandible has been infiltrated. Nonetheless, the cancer principles of a defined resection, as documented anew by Looser et al. [15], must be strictly observed from the viewpoint of curative therapy in both enoral and transoral, minimally invasive and function-conserving operative techniques.

Based on our reported results we also emphasize that enoral/transoral management of malignancies of the oral cavity and the oropharynx is a promising oncological concept causing less discomfort and impairment for the patients. In our opinion a decisive precondition for the enoral/transoral approach to the tumor is that it is recognized and seen in its borders, i.e. the tumor must be sufficiently exposed during operation. Tumor expansion into the soft tissues of the neck, reaching the internal jugular vein or the carotid artery is seen as a contraindication for enoral/transoral tumor resection. In these cases or if the malignancies have infiltrated larger parts of bony structures, e.g. the mandible, a modified approach from outside with reconstruction of defects – if necessary – by predicled or microvasculary anastomosed flaps is recommended.

References

1   Martin H, Sugerbaker EL: Cancer of the tonsil. Am J Surg 1941;52:158–196.
2   Conley JJ, von Fraenkel T: Historical aspect of head and neck surgery. Ann Otol 1956;65: 643–655.
3   UICC: TNM Classification of Malignant Tumours, ed 4. Berlin, Springer, 1987.
4   Barrs DM, DeSanto LW, O'Fallon WM: Squamous cell carcinoma of the tonsil and tongue-base region. Arch Otolaryngol 1979;105:479–485.
5   Frame JW, Morgan D, Rhys Evans PH: Tongue resection with the CO_2 laser: The effects of past radiotherapy on postoperative complications. Br J Oral Maxillofac Surg 1988;26:464–471.
6   Marks JE, Lee F, Freeman RB, Zivnuska FR: Carcinoma of the oral tongue: A study of patient selection and treatment results. Laryngoscope 1981;91:1548–1559.
7   Panje WR, Scher N, Karnell M: Transoral carbon dioxide laser ablation for cancer, tumors, and other diseases. Arch Otolaryngol Head Neck Surg 1989;115:681–688.
8   Rhys Williams S, Carruth JAS: The role of the carbon dioxide laser in treatment of carcinoma of the tongue. J Laryngol Otol 1988;102:1122–1123.
9   Strong E: Surgical management of oral cancer. Dent Clin North Am 1990;34:185–203.
10 Jahnke V: Die Chirurgie der Zungen- und Mundbodentumoren. Arch Ohren-Nasen-Kehlkopf-heilkd 1975;210:275.
11 Meyer H-J, Terrahe K, Haug H, Schmidt W: Die freie Dünndarmtransplantation zur plastischen Rekonstruktion von Mundhöhle, Pharynx und zervikalem Ösophagus. Laryngol Rhinol Otol 1988;67:1–6.

12   Rudert H: Die chirurgische Behandlung der Oropharynxtumoren. Arch Otorhinolaryngol 1984;241(suppl II):92–102.
13   Steiner W: Endoscopic therapy of early laryngeal cancer. Indications and results; Wigand ME, Steiner W, Stell PM (eds): Functional Partial Laryngectomy. Conservation Surgery for Carcinoma of the Larynx. Berlin, Springer, 1984, pp 163–170.
14   Denecke HJ: Die oto-rhino-laryngologischen Operationen; in Kirschner M, Guleke ZN, Zenker R (eds): Allgemeine und Spezielle Chirurgische Operationslehre, ed 2. Berlin, Springer, 1953, vol 5, pp 286–294.
15   Looser KG, Shah JP, Strong EW: The significance of 'positive' margins in surgically resected epidermoid carcinomas. Head Neck Surg 1978;1:107.

Priv.-Doz. Dr. H. Iro, Department of Oto-Rhino-Laryngology, Head and Neck Surgery, Waldstrasse 1, D–91045 Erlangen (Germany)

Rudert H, Werner JA (eds): Lasers in Otorhinolaryngology, and in Head and Neck Surgery.
Adv Otorhinolaryngol. Basel, Karger, 1995, vol 49, pp 196–200

....

An Analysis of Recurrences after Transoral Laser Resection of Oral Carcinoma

Hans Edmund Eckel [a], *Walter Franz Thumfart* [b]

[a] Department of Oto-Rhino-Laryngology, University of Cologne, Germany;
[b] Department of Oto-Rhino-Laryngology, University of Innsbruck, Austria

Currently, transoral resection of oral cavity and oropharynx carcinoma is generally believed to be indicated for the treatment of verrucous cancers and small epidermoid carcinomas in the absence of metastatic lymph nodes [1]. However, such treatment is thought to be inadequate for more advanced carcinomas or tumors with clinically positive or suspected occult lymph node metastases. In such advanced disease, an extraoral approach permits excellent exposure of the tumor, en bloc resection of the primary with the regional lymph nodes and the intervening lymphatics, and immediate reconstruction of the surgical defect [2, 3]. Recently, transoral laser surgery has been reported to provide a safe and reliable alternative to extraoral surgery [4–9]. Only limited and controversial data on this concept have been published so far [10, 11]. This paper focuses on the patterns and treatment of recurrences after laser surgery for oral carcinoma to provide additional information on the appropriate choice of surgical treatment.

Patients and Methods

One hundred and seventeen patients with infiltrating oral carcinoma were treated for cure with transoral resection of the primary and staged neck dissection. Patient characteristics are given in table 1. All patients were followed up for 3–7 years from the initiation of tumor-directed therapy unless they died. The data on absolute and adjusted survival of these patients are given in detail in the article 'Transoral laser surgery for oral carcinoma' [this vol., pp. 185–190]. The data of all patients were prospectively collected in a database including information on the patterns of recurrences observed after the onset of primary treatment. These data were evaluated for this investigation.

Table 1. Patient characteristics and staging (TNM) of 117 patients with infiltrating oral cavity and oropharynx carcinoma

Age	28–85 (median 56)			
Sex	28 F 89 M			
Performance status	0–2 (WHO)			
Site	oral cavity: 64 oropharynx: 53			
TNM stage	T 1 N 0: 22	T 1 N 1: 4	T 1 N 2: 3	T 1 N 3: –
	T 2 N 0: 41	T 2 N 1: 6	T 2 N 2: 2	T 2 N 3: 1
	T 3 N 0: 17	T 3 N 1: 9	T 3 N 2: 7	T 3 N 3: 2
	T 4 N 0: 1	T 4 N 1: 1	T 4 N 2: –	T 4 N 3: 1

Results

The obtained specimen showed occult metastases in 17 patients, i.e. in 17% of the patients with clinically negative neck. Forty-seven recidives were diagnosed during the follow-up period. Four of the recurrences were isolated in the neck with no evidence of recurrence at the site of the primary. These 4 patients were salvaged by performing a neck dissection on a previously untreated contralateral neck or by resection of isolated regional metastases. Thirteen patients eventually developed recurrences at the site of the primary alone, and 28 patients at the site of the primary and in the neck. In 6 of these patients, a second transoral laser resection was performed, and 6 patients had radical extraoral salvage surgery. The remaining 29 had radiotherapy or palliative symptomatic therapy only. Two patients died of distant metastases with no evidence of local or regional recurrence. Tables 2 and 3 demonstrate the number of recidives and deaths as related to the site of the primary and to TNM classification of the tumors.

Discussion

The value of transoral laser resection of early oral carcinoma has been demonstrated repeatedly over the past 15 years [4, 6–8]. Nagorsky and Sessions [12] reported a 77% local control rate following laser resection or early and locally advanced oral cavity cancer (T1–3 N0) in 28 patients with clinically negative neck. No surgical treatment of the neck was performed.

Table 2. Outcome of 117 patients with oral carcinoma as related to the site of primary tumor

Primary	n	Recurrences		Deceased	
		n	%	n	%
Oral cavity					
Anterior 2/3 of tongue	34	9	26	7	21
Floor of the mouth	24	10	42	8	33
Alveolar ridge (mandible)	1	0	0	0	0
Buccal cavity	4	4	100	3	75
Retromolar triangle	1	0	0	0	0
Total	64	23	36	18	28
Oropharynx					
Soft palate and uvula	17	4	24	4	24
Tonsil	26	12	46	9	35
Posterior wall	2	1	50	1	50
Base of tongue	8	5	62	5	62
Total	53	22	42	19	36
All patients	117	45	38	37	32

The results published in these studies suggest that transoral laser surgery for the treatment of oral carcinoma leads to good local control rates and to excellent functional results, but do not focus on the problem of regional lymph node metastases that are frequently encountered in oral carcinoma. Laser surgery was only performed in patients in whom lymph node metastases were not suspected, or radiotherapy was chosen to treat the neck following transoral removal of the primary.

It is, however, well known that neck metastases are frequently to be found in patients with carcinoma of the oral cavity or oropharynx. Decroix and Ghossein [13] reported that 219 (36%) of 602 unselected patients with cancer of the tongue had clinical evidence of nodal involvement. Brennan et al. [14], more recently, found clinically obvious neck metastases in 115 (51%) of 224 unselected patients with carcinoma of the oropharynx. But even in the absence of suspect lymph nodes by the time of tumor diagnosis, there is a high risk for occult, subclinical metastases. These will progress to regional recurrence of the disease if the neck remains untreated and therapy focuses on the elimination of the primary only. Bradfield and Scruggs [15] found occult cervical node metastasis in an elective neck dissection or subsequent neck recurrence in an in-

Table 3. Outcome of 117 patients with oral carcinoma as related to TNM classification

Stage	n	Recurrences		Deceased	
		n	%	n	%
T1N0	22	3	14	2	9
T1N1–3	7	2	29	2	29
T2N0	41	11	27	9	22
T2N1–3	9	5	56	4	44
T3N0	17	7	41	5	29
T3N1–3	18	14	78	13	72
T4N0	1	1	100	0	0
T4N1–3	2	2	100	2	100
All patients	117	45	38	37	32

itially negative neck in 14.5% (9/62) of patients with carcinoma of the mobile tongue staged T1N0 and in 30.6% (11/36) of patients staged T2 N0. Fu and co-workers observed subsequent cervical lymph node metastases in 20% of 105 patients with carcinoma of the floor of mouth (51 T1N0, 42 T2N0 and 12 T3N0) treated mainly with radiotherapy or local excision of the tumor. De-croix and Ghossein [13] reported occult metastases in 34% of the neck dissection specimen of 244 patients with cancer of the tongue stages T1–3N0.

While the application of laser surgery has greatly contributed to transoral surgical techniques, it is obviously not suited for the treatment of cervical neck nodes. Additional therapy options are therefore necessary.

Although the oncological data presented in this study were gained from a selected group of patients and follow-up is at present only available for a period of 3 or more years, they strongly suggest that the concept described here is as safe as the traditional surgical concepts. However, infiltrating tumors of the buccal mucosa had a very poor outcome in this series. The small number of patients presenting with this localisation of primary permits no final decision on whether these may better be excluded from transoral resection.

References

1   Schuller DE: Use of the laser in the oral cavity. Otolaryngol Clin North Am 1990;23:31–42.
2   Strong EW: Carcinoma of the tongue. Otolaryngol Clin North Am 1979;12:107–114.
3   Shaha AR, Spiro RH, Shah JP, Strong EW: Squamous carcinoma of the floor of the mouth. Am J Surg 1984;148:456–459.

4   Strong MS, Vaughan CW, Healy GB, Shapshay SM, Jako GJ: Transoral management of local-
    ized carcinoma of the oral cavity using the CO_2 laser. Laryngoscope 1979;89:897–905.
5   Guerry TL, Silverman S, Dedo HH: Carbon dioxide laser resection of superficial oral carci-
    noma: Indications, technique, and results. Ann Otol Rhinol Laryngol 1986;95:547–555.
6   Panje WR, Scher N, Karnell M: Transoral carbon dioxide laser ablation for cancer, tumors, and
    other diseases. Arch Otolaryngol Head Neck Surg 1989;115:681–688.
7   Hirano M, Ohkubo H, Kurita S, Maeda T, Kamimura M, Kawaguchi T, Watanabe Y: CO_2 laser
    in treating carcinoma of the tongue. Auris Nasus Larynx 1985;12:10–14.
8   Steiner W, Aurbach G, Ambrosch P: Minimally invasive therapy in otorhinolaryngology and
    head and neck surgery. Minim Invas Ther 1991;1:57–70.
9   Steiner W: Experience in endoscopic laser surgery of malignant tumours of the upper aero-di-
    gestive tract. Adv Otorhinolaryngol. Basel, Karger, 1988, vol 39, pp 135–144.
10 Leemans CR, Tiwari R, Nauta JJP, Snow GB: Discontinuous vs. incontinuity neck dissection in
    carcinoma of the oral cavity. Arch Otolaryngol Head Neck Surg 1991;117:1003–1006.
11 Spiro RH, Strong EW: Discontinuous partial glossectomy and radical neck dissection in se-
    lected patients with epidermoid carcinoma of the mobile tongue. Am J Surg 1973;126:544–546.
12 Nagorsky MJ, Sessions DG: Laser resection for early oral cavity cancer. Ann Otol Rhinol
    Laryngol 1987;96:556–560.
13 Decroix Y, Ghossein NA: Experience of the Curie Institute in treatment of cancer of the mo-
    bile tongue. Cancer 1981;47:496–508.
14 Brennan CT, Sessions DG, Spitznagel EL Jr, Harvey JE: Surgical pathology of cancer of the
    oral cavity and oropharynx. Laryngoscope 1991;101:1175–1197.
15 Bradfield JS, Scruggs RP: Carcinoma of the mobile tongue: Incidence of cervical metastases in
    early lesions related to method of primary treatment. Laryngoscope 1983;93:1332–1336.

Dr. H.E. Eckel, Universitäts-Hals-Nasen-Ohrenklinik, Joseph-Stelzmann-Strasse 9,
D–50937 Köln (Germany)

Rudert H, Werner JA (eds): Lasers in Otorhinolaryngology, and in Head and Neck Surgery.
Adv Otorhinolaryngol. Basel, Karger, 1995, vol 49, pp 201–206

....

Functional and Clinical Anatomy of the Anterior Commissure

B. Tillmann, F. Paulsen [1]

Anatomisches Institut der Universität Kiel, Germany

The laryngeal anterior commissure includes all structures of the insertion of the vocal ligaments and vocalis muscles as well as the cartilaginous or bony thyroidal skeleton and its mucosa (fig. 1a). The present morphological investigation tries to draw a conclusion on the biomechanical behavior of the insertion from its structure. From a clinical point of view we will demonstrate how the structure of the anterior commissure influences the spread of carcinomas.

Material and Methods

For light microscopy 21 larynges (10 male, 11 female, aged 8–88 years) were embedded in paraffine after fixation in 3% formalin solution and decalcification. Horizontal sections (10 µm) were stained with toluidine-blue (pH 1), resorcinfuchsine-thiazinered-picrinic acid, orceine, azan and according to Masson-Goldner.

Electron microscopy was performed in 29 larynges (18 male, 11 female, aged 35–88 years). Fixation in 3% glutaraldehyde is followed by decalcification and embedding in araldit. Semithin sections are prepared for light microscopy, thin sections for electron microscopy (Zeiss TEM 902).

Immunohistochemical investigations are performed on cryosections of unfixed material (3 male, 3 female, aged 39–87 years), that was frozen at –80 °C. Polyclonal antibodies against collagen type I–III are used.

The insertion of the vocal ligaments in the anterior commissure is investigated with a magnifying glass in six macerated male thyroidal skeletons.

[1] We would like to thank R. Worm and G.R. Klaws for their technical assistance.

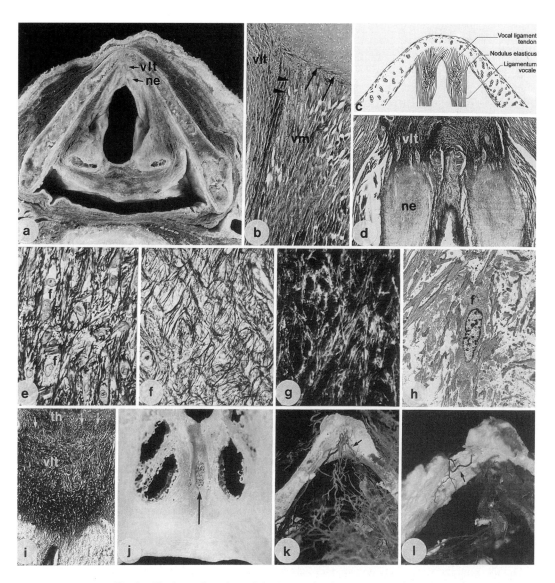

Fig. 1. a Horizontal section of the larynx (male, age 87 years) at the level of the plicae vocales. Noduli elastici (ne) and vocal ligament tendons (vlt) are visible in the anterior commissure. *b* Histological horizontal section of the larynx (male, age 8 years). Vocalis muscle (vm) inserts with medial fibres at vocal ligament tendon (vlt) (arrowheads). The major part of the muscle inserts at the perichondrium (arrows). Masson-Goldner. ×37. *c* Insertion of the vocal ligament at the thyroid. *d* Histological horizontal section of the insertion of the vocal ligament at the anterior commissure (male, age 8 years). ne = Nodulus elasticus; vlt = vocal ligament tendon. Gomori. ×25. *e, f* Histological horizontal sections of nodulus elasticus. *e* Fibroblast-like cells (f) are surrounded by a meshwork

The blood supply of the anterior commissure is investigated by means of arterial injections. The areas supplied by carotid and subclavian arteries are filled with plastic of different colors (corrosion technique [1]).

The presence of blood vessels was investigated with immunohistochemical methods using an antibody against laminin, a component of the basement membrane.

Results

The vocalis muscle (fig. 1b) inserts at perichondrium or periosteum in the anterior commissure of the thyroidal skeleton mainly with short tendons. Muscle fibres of the medial aspect become part of the vocal ligament tendon.

The vocal ligament inserts at the thyroidal skeleton with two characteristic structures (fig. 1c, d): In front of the insertion in the anterior commissure noduli elastici are embedded in the ventral part of the vocal ligaments. The ligaments insert via tendons.

Extracellular matrix of the noduli elastici consists of reticular and elastic fibres that are interwoven especially in the medial aspect. The fibres are organized as a meshwork around embedded cells (fig. 1e, f). The ultrastructure of these embedded cells equals the appearance of fibroblasts in electron microscopy (fig. 1h). In the lateral aspect of the nodulus elasticus, the fibres are less mixed than in the medial part. Immunohistochemistry confirms the presence of type III collagen in nodulus elasticus (fig. 1g), there is no type I collagen. Reticular fibres from nodulus elasticus become part of the vocal ligament tendon and partly cross over to the opposite side. The vocal ligament tendon consists of a dense network of fibres that mix in horizontal and vertical direction (fig. 1i). These fibres derive from the vocal ligament, conus elasticus, the medial aspect of the vocalis tendon and the quadrangular membrane. Light microscpy demonstrates collagenous, reticular and elastic fibres. Immunohistochemical staining shows the presence of type I and type III collagen.

of fibres (male, age 57 years). Toluidine blue. × 320. *f* Staining according to Gomori (male, age 48 years) demonstrates the meshwork of reticular fibres. × 320. *g* Immuno histochemical staining of type III collagen. The distribution of fibres equals the course of the reticular fibres. × 320. *h* Electron microscopy (male, age 51 years) of a fibroblast (f) surrounded by elastic fibres and collagenous fibrils. × 1160. *i* Histological horizontal section of vocal ligament tendon (vlt) (male, age 8 years). The fibres are interwoven in horizontal and vertical directions. In the area of insertion (arrows) at the thyroid cartilage (th) perichondrium is absent. Gomori. × 30. *j* Bony skeleton of a macerated thyroid (male, age 77 years). The bony surface at the insertion of the vocal ligament is roughened and shows neat perforations (arrow). *k, l* Corrosion preparation of the laryngeal arteries filled with plastic. *k* Arteries of plica vocalis heading towards the anterior commissure (arrow). *l* Thin vessels enter the bony laryngeal skeleton (arrow).

In the cartilaginous thyroidal skeleton collagenous fibres directly pass over to the hyaline cartilage. In the area of insertion of the vocal ligament tendon no perichondrium or periosteum is to be found. The extracellular matrix of the area of insertion of the vocal ligaments shows a marked positive reaction when stained with toluidine blue.

In some ossified thyroidal cartilage skeletons, a small zone of hyaline cartilage is visible in the area of insertion of the vocal ligament at the bony skeleton. In completely ossified thyroidal cartilage skeletons chondroid cells are embedded in the vocal ligament tendon in this area.

In the macerated ossified thyroidal skeleton the area of insertion of the vocal ligament is clearly visible with a magnifying glass (fig. 1j). The bony surface of this area is roughened, small perforations that connect to the bone below are visible.

Arterial injection of plastic can demonstrate the blood supply of larynx in corrosion samples (fig. 1h, e). In plica vocalis, which is mainly supplied by the superior laryngeal artery, small arteries pass over to the anterior commissure. In the ossified thyroidal skeleton vessels can be followed into the bone in the area of the anterior commissure. Light microscopy shows vessels that enter the bone in the area of insertion of the vocal ligament. The arteries of the anterior commissure are connected with extralaryngeal vessels that derive from the cricothyroidal branch. Light microscopy and immunohistochemistry demonstrate a complete absence of blood vessels in the cartilaginous skeleton of the anterior commissure.

Discussion

The structures of the anterior commissure, resembling the insertion of vocalis muscle and vocal ligament, have to fulfill biomechanical functions. Comparable to tendinous insertions at the limbs, differently structured areas of insertion are visible in the larynx as well [2, 3]. The tendinous insertions of the skeleton of trunk and limbs are classified according to their histological structure in chondro-apophyseal and periostal-diaphyseal insertions [4–6]. It is the function of the extracellular matrix to equalize the different elastic modules of tendon and skeleton.

Vocalis muscle inserts via perichondrium or periosteum and is comparable to periosteal-diaphyseal tendinous insertions. Force is transmitted between skeleton and tendon over a great surface, due to the spread insertion of the tendinous tissue via perichondrium or periosteum.

Two structures are integrated in the insertion of the vocal ligament that contribute to the equalization of different elastic modules [3]. Inside the nodulus elasticus the meshwork of elastic and reticular fibres together with embedded cells leads to a decrease of transverse shortening of the tissue. Due to this mechanism longitudinal extension of the vocal ligament is decreased in the area of insertion which results in a lowered extension of the tissue.

The connective tissue between noduli elastici and the thyroidal skeleton occasionally is called Broyles' tendon after a description of the laryngologist Edwin Broyles [7] although the structure of the vocal ligament tendon was already described in the 19th century by von Luschka [8], Fränkel [9] and Reinke [10]. Schumacher [11] introduced the term 'Faserwulst', giving the most sufficient description of the tissue as a bulge of fibres.

The functional adaptation of the vocal ligament tendon functions by the order of its fibres and due to its richness in acidic glycosaminoglycans. Vocal ligament tendon is mechanically comparable to chondro-apophyseal tendinous insertions.

The structures of the vocal ligaments insertion at the thyroid cartilage are of high clinical importance considering the spread of carcinomas which can extend along vocal ligament tendon to the skeleton of the thyroid cartilage [7, 12]. The vocal ligament tendon does not seem to be a barrier as described by Kirchner and Carter [13]. Absence of perichondrium and connective tissue fibres attached to the skeleton promote the growth of tumors in a ventral direction. An important factor for the invasion of tumors is ossification of the thyroid cartilage and the associated vascularization of the Thyroidal skeleton [14]. Intralaryngeal vessels of the anterior commissure connect via the skeleton with extralaryngeal vessels. It could well be that these vessels and associated lymphatics, apart from those that pass through the cricothyroideal ligament, play an important role in the rare spread to prelaryngeal lymph nodes.

References

1   Claassen H, Klaws GR: Preparation of four-color arterial corrosion casts of the laryngeal arteries. Surg Radiol Anat 1992;14:301–305.
2   Fischer M, Tillmann B: Tendinous insertions in the human thyroid cartilage plate: macroscopic and histologic studies. Anat Embryol 1991;183:251–257.
3   Tillmann B, Schünke M: Untersuchungen zur Struktur der Plica vocalis des Menschen. Arch Ohr-Nas-Kehlkopfheilk 1989;(suppl II):11–18.
4   Petersen H: Die Organe des Skelettsystems; in von Möllendorff W (ed): Handbuch der mikroskopischen Anatomie des Menschen. Berlin, Springer, 1930, pp 521–678.
5   Biermann H: Die Knochenbildung im Bereich periostaler-diaphysärer Sehnen- und Bandansätze. Z Zellforsch 1957;46:635–671.
6   Knese KH, Biermann H: Die Knochenbildung an Sehnen- und Bandansätzen im Bereich ursprünglich chondraler Apophysen. Z Zellforsch 1958;49:142–187.
7   Broyles E: The anterior commissure tendon. Ann Otol Rhinol Laryngol 1943;52:342–345.
8   von Luschka H: Der Kehlkopf des Menschen. Tübingen, Laupp, 1871.

9   Fränkel B: Studien zur feineren Anatomie des Kehlkopfes. Arch Laryngol 1894;1:1–24.
10 Reinke F: Über die funktionelle Struktur der menschlichen Stimmlippe. Mit besonderer Berücksichtigung des elastischen Gewebes. Anat Hefte 1897;9:104–115.
11 Schumacher S: Histologie des Kehlkopfes; in Denker, Kahler (eds): Handbuch der Hals-Nasen-Ohren-Heilkunde. Berlin, Springer, 1925, vol 1.
12 Olofsson J: Glottic carcinoma – with special reference to tumors involving the anterior commissure and subglottis; in Wiegand ME, Steiner W, Stell PM (eds): Functional Partial Laryngectomy: Conservation Surgery for Carcinoma of the Larynx. Berlin, Springer, 1984, pp 131–134.
13 Kirchner JA, Carter D: Intralaryngeal barriers to the spread of cancer. Acta Otolaryngol (Stockh) 1987;103:503–513.
14 Andrea M: Vasculature of the anterior commissure. Ann Otol Rhinol Laryngol 1981;90:18–20.

Prof. Dr. med. Bernhard Tillmann, Anatomisches Institut der Universität Kiel,
Olshausenstrasse 40, D-24098 Kiel (Germany)

Rudert H, Werner JA (eds): Lasers in Otorhinolaryngology, and in Head and Neck Surgery.
Adv Otorhinolaryngol. Basel, Karger, 1995, vol 49, pp 207–211

··

Imaging in Advanced Laryngeal Cancer before Laser Surgery

A Critical Review

Joachim Schubert, Martin Heller

Klinik für Radiologische Diagnostik, Christian-Albrecht-Universität Kiel,
Deutschland

Indications for and limits of laser surgery are still under discussion. Imaging may help decide between a laser surgical approach and more radical conventional procedures like laryngectomy.

In most cases, the diagnosis of a malignant tumor is made by clinical assessment and histologic examination. Aims of imaging are definition of the local tumor stage, detection of involved lymph nodes and eventually distant metastases.

Prior to laser surgery, the surgeon needs information about tumor extent, including: (a) infiltration in the anterior commissure; (b) involvement of the supralaryngeal space, e.g. preepiglottic space and tongue base; (c) infiltration of the thyroid cartilage; (d) infiltration of cricoid or arytenoid cartilages; (e) penetration of the cricothyreoid membrane.

Methods

The most important methods today are CT and MRI. Superior soft tissue contrast, visibility of the deep and paralaryngeal regions and in case of MRI multiplanar imaging renders them the methods of choice. Only these methods will be discussed.

Ultrasonography is not able to assess the cartilage and the partially airfilled spaces of the larynx.

Angiography is sometimes done to detect vascular invasion in widespread tumors.

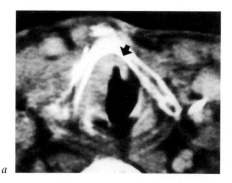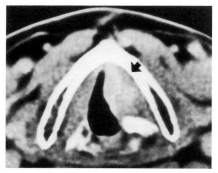

a　　　　　　　　　　　　　　　　　　　　　　　　　　　　　　　　　　　　*b*

Fig. 1.a CT scan. True cord tumor on the right side with spread through the anterior commissure (arrow). *b* CT scan at true cord level. Bulky left-sided glottic cancer (arrow) makes evaluation of the anterior commissure difficult.

Technique

CT. CT in laryngeal cancer is done as thin slice CT with 1.5–3 mm slice thickness. 1.5–2 mm slices allow better differentiation of small structures. The administered doses of contrast agent range from 100 to 200 ml (300 mg iodine/ml), a precontrast study is not routinely recommended.

For evaluation of the anterior commissure, scanning should be obtained in quiet breathing to keep vocal cords abducted. To show the piriform recessus and (if tumor involved) the free epiglottis, a functional image of these regions with e-phonation or modified valsalva-maneuver may be added.

MRI. Transversal spin density- and T2-weighted series in spin echo technique and T1-weighted images in sagittal, transverse and coronal orientation are generally obtained. After i.v. Gadolineum DTPA, the T1-weighted scans in at least 2 orientations are repeated. Slice thickness depends on technical facilities; most common are 3–4 mm for T1-weighted and 5 mm for spin density/T2-weighted images. There is discussion whether T1 images should be rather obtained with the spin echo or gradient echo technique; by now, most authors prefer spin echo sequences.

Anterior Commissure

In CT, absence of tumor spread in the anterior commissure is easy to evaluate if there is no soft tissue visible. Every detection of soft tissue is suspect, if vocal cords are regularly abducted (fig. 1a). However, differentiation between tumor, edema and inflammatory changes might be difficult. Contrast enhancement may occur in all these conditions. Also in conditions with fixation of the vocal cord or a large, bulky vocal cord tumor evaluation is less specific (fig. 1b).

MRI seems to have no advantage in these problems; with common limitations in image quality due to artifacts, it can be markedly inferior to CT.

Supraglottic Spread

The preepiglottic space is clearly visible by the characteristic appearance of fatty tissue both on CT and MRI scans. Also, thickening of the epiglottis can be detected with both methods. If it is uncertain if the tumor is a supraglottic laryngeal cancer or a hypopharynx carcinoma arising from the piriform sinus, CT with modified Valsalva maneuver spreads the piriform sinus and so may lead to differentiation.

The ventricle is not visible in CT as it is parallel to the axial slices. Here MRI has the important advantage of coronal imaging. Even if the ventricle has collapsed because of a bulky true cord tumor, the fat signal of the false chord reaching the thyroid cartilage in normal configuration makes infiltration unlikely. Involvement of the base of the tongue is also better visible on sagittal MRI than on axial CT planes.

Thyroid Cartilage Invasion

CT shows invasion or destruction very well, if the cartilage is homogeneously calcified. This, however, is not the case in most subjects. In inhomogeneously calcified cartilage, only larger destructions are detectable. Although noncalcified cartilage is more resistant against infiltration, distinction to tumor invasion may be impossible in CT. In MRI, tumor tissue appears with higher signal on spin density images, while noncalcified cartilage generally has low signal intensity. This advantage counts only in case of good image quality.

Arytenoid or Cricoid Cartilage Invasion

Infiltration of the arytenoid cartilage is to be suspected if the cartilage is partly surrounded by tumor tissue. Destruction or sclerotic changes are direct signs of infiltration (fig. 2). The criteria of cricoid involvement are similar to those in thyroid cartilage evaluation.

Assessment of the cricoarytenoid region is more difficult due to its complex structure. Compared with the thyroid cartilage, the results of imaging procedures are inferior. MRI with multiplanar imaging seems to have advantages.

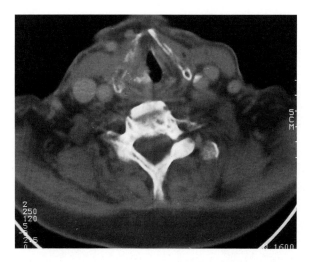

Fig. 2. CT scan at ventricle/true cord level. Destruction of the thyroid cartilage by right-sided glottic cancer (arrow). Incomplete calcification also on the left side. Sclerosis of the right arytenoid cartilage indicates infiltration (arrowhead).

Spread through the Cricothyreoid Membrane

Although the conus elasticus mostly cannot be identified on CT and MRI images as a different structure, tumor spread through it can be seen as atypical soft tissue in the anterior cervical region. There is no definite difference in performance between CT and MRI in this respect.

How Reliable Are the Results of Imaging?

During the last years, several studies compared the results of imaging and pathological studies [1–4]. The majority of the reported results for correct T staging (as far as possible with imaging) are between 70 and 90%, generally with an advantage of some percentage points for MRI [7]. For most questions listed in the preceding sections, further differentiation is not possible because case numbers are too small. There are two important reservations:

(1) Castelijns et al. [1] found a sensitivity for cartilage invasion in CT of only 46 vs. 89% in MRI particularly because of very poor results in arytenoid and cricoid evaluation.

(2) Nearly all studies comparing CT and MRI results do not list the number of patients excluded because of nondiagnostic MRI images due to gross

motion artifacts. In the study of Castelijns et al. [1], where this fraction is reported, it is 16%.

CT or MRI?

The question, what method should be performed (first) is, next to availability, patient dependent. In a fairly cooperative subject, we would do MRI. If there are still unsolved questions, CT may follow, eventually as functional imaging. Patients in more reduced general condition should undergo CT.

Outlook

CT will be gradually improved by faster scanners with better imaging quality. Especially, thin-slice spiral scanning will be possible with longer scan range and higher density resolution. Todays results, however, are a still somewhat inferior to conventional scanning.

MRI will probably make more significant progress. Most important will be functional imaging. New ultrafast imaging sequences already allow single or few slice imaging during phonation; however, there are no reported results of diagnostic applications to now.

Still an important matter will be communication between clinicians and radiologists. For examination planning with advancing technical abilities, for quality control and for correct interpretation of limited imaging results close contact between the different specialities seems to be essential.

References

1   Castelijns JA, Gerritse GJ, Kaiser MC, Valk J, van Zanten TEG, Golding RG, Meyer CJLM, van Hattum LH, Sprenger M, Bezemer PD, Snow GB: Invasion of laryngeal cartilage by cancer: Comparison of CT and MR imaging. Radiology 1987;166:199–206.
2   Bohndorf W: Beurteilung von Larynxkarzinomen vor Therapie: Wert von Computertomographie und Magnetresonanztomographie. Strahlenther Onkol 1991;167:239–243.
3   Lenz M: Computertomographie und Kernspintomographie bei Kopf-Hals-Tumoren. Stuttgart, Thieme, 1992.
4   Mafee MF, Schild JA, Michael AS, Choi KH, Capek V: Cartilage involvement in laryngeal carcinoma: Correlation of CT and pathologic macrosection studies. J Comp Assist Tomogr 1984;8: 969–973.
5   Steinkamp HJ, Heim T, Mäurer J, Mathe F, Felix R: Wertigkeit von Magnetresonanztomographie und Computertomographie im Tumorstaging des Larynx-/Hypopharynxkarzinoms. RöFo 1993;158, 5:437–444.

Joachim Schubert, Klinik für Radiologische Diagnostik, Christian-Albrecht-Universität Kiel, Arnold-Heller-Strasse 9, D–24105 Kiel (Germany)

Rudert H, Werner JA (eds): Lasers in Otorhinolaryngology, and in Head and Neck Surgery.
Adv Otorhinolaryngol. Basel, Karger, 1995, vol 49, pp 212–214

....

Classification of Endolaryngeal Laser Partial Laryngectomies

Walter Franz Thumfart[a], *Hans Edmund Eckel*[b], *Georg Mathias Sprinzl*[a]

[a] Universitäts-Hals-Nasen-Ohrenklinik Innsbruck
   (Vorstand: Universitätsprof. *W.F. Thumfart*), Innsbruck, Österreich;
[b] Universitäts-Hals-Nasen-Ohrenklinik Köln (Direktor: Universitätsprof. *E. Stennert*),
   Köln, Deutschland

Since the introduction of microlaryngoscopic laser surgery [1], the indication for a transoral endoscopic partial laryngeal resection has been widely modified and expanded by numerous authors. The resection of expansive glottis carcinomas and of subglottic and supraglottic tumors has continued to be the subject of controversy [2–4]. On the one hand, seasoned laryngologists doubt the oncological safety of extensive endolaryngeal resections, and in view of the substantiated safety of endolaryngeal surgery via conventional microinstruments, doubts arise in regard to the usefulness of laser surgery among such carcinomas [5]. On the other hand, various authors have in the meanwhile made assertions indicating that laser-assisted microlaryngoscopic operative procedures have notably increased the indication for endoscopic surgical treatment of glottis and supraglottis carcinomas [3, 4]. Further, the opinion is spreading among well-versed laser surgeons that the majority of all laryngeal carcinomas can be kept in check surgically using this method.

The difficulty of evaluating the value of certain treatment modalities can be lessened by a critical analysis of their flaws. In addition, the analysis of such flaws could allow for the improvement of the planning of operations and techniques [4].

Material and Methods

The authors have developed four different types of endolaryngeal laser resections for the treatment of larynx carcinomas. From 1986 onwards, 204 patients with laryngeal cancers were treated by endoscopic laser surgery. Respective tumor stages were accompanied by a mono- or bilateral elective or curative neck dissections at different points in

Table 1. Laser resection types

	Extension of resection	Type of tumour
Type I	vocal cord mucosa	Tis
Type II	cordectomy, anterior third of the other vocal cord intact	T1a
Type III	extended cordectomy, anterior commissure down to thyroid cartilage, subglottic region including cricothyroid membrane	T1b
Type IV	laryngeal exenteration, all endolaryngeal structures down to thyroid and cricoid cartilages and arytaenoid cartilage	T2

time; this applies to 45 patients, 19 of which displayed lymph node metastases. Both these and the majority of the patients with supraglottic carcinomas were subsequently subjected to radiation therapy after their respective surgical treatments. Patients among which palliative procedures were performed or among which a primary laser resection was not possible within healthy margins and who thus required further transcollar operations were not included in this examination.

The clinical data of all 204 patients are registered in a databank. The databank contains information concerning the anatomical location of the primary tumor, the histological tumor diagnosis and the treatment applied. The posttherapeutic status is documented as based on the findings made in the follow-up treatment in the tumor consultation sessions of the clinic or those findings derived from colleagues elsewhere. If a tumor recidivation was diagnosed, the date, location and expanse of the recidivation as well as the required treatment were all documented.

Twenty laryngectomy specimens were plastinated [6] and reduced to whole-organ sectional series. By means of such whole-organ sections, the growth of laryngeal tumors was well determinable [7, 8]. Based on these data, the locoregional recidivations were placed into the following categories: 'anterior commissure', 'vocal cord', 'arytenoid cartilage', 'transglottic region', 'base of the tongue or supraglottic structures' and 'lymph nodes of the neck'. The evaluation of these data was performed with the goal of locating the most common anatomical sites of recidivation.

Results

The present inidations for laser surgery of larynx carcinomas are glottic carcinomas, as well as supraglottic and subglottic carcinomas up to stage T2. Table 1 present the different types of resection in our endolaryngeal laser laryngectomy concept.

Laser surgery is an effective approach to the curative treatment of T1 and T2 tumors of the glottis and of individual cases of subglottic and supraglottic tumors of the larynx. The classification of endolaryngeal laser partial laryngectomies and the follow-up of the patients treated this method shows that deeply infiltrating tumors in the region of the anterior commissure can not steadily be removed by transoral laser surgery. The following projects on development of transoral laser surgery procedures must aim at the complete transoral resection of the anterior part of the thyroid or at least achieve thermal sterilization of this area.

Discussion

Although in our own collective a supraglottic expanse of recidivations was only viewed as an exception in one case, our findings do support the observations of Kleinsasser [8] that tumor recidivations in the region of the anterior commissure often extend into the subglottic space and to the ligamentum cricothyreoideum; from there they often infiltrate the laryngeal skeleton towards the surface and can continue to spread into the thyroid gland.

This subglottic direction of expansion of carcinomas of the anterior commissure is therefore assigned its own operation type III – for carcinomas of the anterior commissure T1b – and IV – for transglottic carcinomas – endolaryngeal partial larynx resections, as the subglottic inner anterior laryngeal cartilage perichondrium and the membrana cricothyroidea are included in the resection in this operation [2, 5].

It is reasonable to define different types of resections, because different types of tumors require different kinds of surgical procedures. These different procedures will probably lead to better individual anatomic and functional results [2].

References

1   Strong MS, Jako GJ: Laser surgery in the larynx. Early clinical experiences with continuous CO_2 laser. Ann Otol 1972;81:791–798.
2   Eckel HE, Thumfart WF: Laser surgery for the treatment of larynx carcinoma. Indications, techniques and preliminary results. Ann Otol Rhinol Laryngol 1992;101:113–118.
3   Rudert H: Larynx- und Hypopharynxkarzinome – Endoskopische Chirurgie mit dem Laser: Möglichkeiten und Grenzen. Arch Oto-Rhino-Laryngol 1991;(suppl 1):3–18.
4   Steiner W: Experience in endoscopic laser surgery of malignant tumours of the upper aero-digestive tract. Adv Otorhinolaryngol. Basel, Karger, 1988, vol 39, pp 135–144.
5   Thumfart WF, Eckel HE: Endolaryngeale Laser-Chirurgie zur Behandlung von Kehlkopfkarzinomen. Das aktuelle Kölner-Konzept. HNO 1990;38:174–178.
6   Eckel HE, Sittel CH, Sprinzl GM, Walger M, Koebke J: Plastination: A new approach to morphological research and instruction with excised larynges. Trans Am Laryngol Assoc 1993;in press.
7   Kirchner JA: Cancer at the anterior commissure of the larynx. Arch Otolaryngol 1970;91: 524–525.
8   Kleinsasser O: Mikrolaryngoskopie und endolaryngeale Mikrochirurgie, Aufl. 3. Stuttgart, Schattauer, 1991.

Univ.-Prof. Dr. Dr. med. Walter Franz Thumfart, Universitäts-Hals-Nasen-Ohrenklinik, Anichstrasse 35, A–6020 Innsbruck (Austria)

Rudert H, Werner JA (eds): Lasers in Otorhinolaryngology, and in Head and Neck Surgery.
Adv Otorhinolaryngol. Basel, Karger, 1995, vol 49, pp 215–218

....

Phonatory Ability after Surgery of Vocal Cord Carcinoma of Limited Extension

A Comparison between Transoral Laser Microsurgery and Frontolateral Partial Laryngeal Resection

Ulrich Reker

Phoniatry at the Department of Otorhinolaryngology, Head and Neck Surgery,
University of Kiel, Germany

For the choice of the mode of treatment of vocal cord carcinoma the curative rate is the most important factor to be considered. But the factor of post-treatment phonatory ability and voice quality should also be considered. This especially, as consciousness of the patients for the restrictions by his dysphonia is growing considerably. This goes so far that in some countries radiation therapy with its good voice results is preferred to surgery. In the opinion of the author, it will in the long term be necessary to inform the patient that radiation therapy with good voice results is possible, though there are other substantial disadvantages.

Postoperative phonatory ability after different surgical forms of treatment of vocal cord carcinoma is very rarely examined scientifically and from a phoniatric point of view. The development of modern phoniatric methods makes it possible to examine vocal ability not only psychoacoustically, but also objectively, using different methods to reach the necessary multidimensional approach to describe phonatory ability.

We examined 21 patients who had an endoscopic laser cordectomy and 33 patients who had conventional surgery in the form of a frontolateral partial larynx resection. Both groups were examined at least half a year after surgery. There was no sign of recurrence.

Table 1 shows details of laryngoscopic and stroboscopic findings. The fact that partial larynx resection had a higher number of T1b tumors in respect to the laser group, does not allow statistic comparison. Nevertheless, there is a fundamental difference in stroboscopic and laryngoscopic findings:

Table 1. Stroboscopic and laryngoscopic findings after treatment of vocal fold carcinoma

	Laser (n = 21)	Partial resection (n = 33)
Mobility of cricoarytenoid articulation		
Normal	20	8
Reduced	1	16
Missing	–	9
Glottal closure with phonation		
No gap or <1 mm	5	1
Gap <2.5 mm	9	5
Gap >2.5 mm	7	26
Pseudo vocal fold		
Large	12	3
Small	7	21
Missing	2	9
Vibration of pseudo vocal fold (mucosal wave)		
Normal	–	–
Reduced	3	–
Missing	18	33

Laser group: 21 patients; mean follow-up 29.6 months; minimum: 6 months. Staging: Tis = 2, T1a = 16, T1b = 1, T2 = 1, T3 = 1.

Frontolateral partial larynx resection: 33 Patients; mean follow-up 46 months; minimum: 6 months. Staging: T1a = 21, T1b = 8, T2 = 4.

(a) The mobility of the crico-arytenoid articulation is nearly always normal (in 20 of all 21 patients) after laser resection, while after partial resection it was normal in only 8 of the 33 patients.

(b) Glottal closure with phonation after laser resection was mostly acceptable. However, after conventional resection, 26 of the 33 patients showed a gap of more than 2.5 mm during phonation.

Figure 1 shows a very favorable example of the development of the thick pseudo vocal fold after partial laser cordectomy. Despite resection, the cicatric pseudo vocal cord is thicker than the healthy vocal fold. Thus, a complete glottal closure with phonation results. However, it has to be reminded that the cicatric pseudo vocal fold after laser resection has practically no vibratory quality if the laser resection goes beyond an exclusively mucosal resection. If part of the vocalis muscle has to be resected, a nonvibrating vocal fold of satisfactory thickness will generally result, but the vibratory pattern of a healthy vocal fold (mucosal wave) is not present. Correspondingly, the voice is always rough and in some way limited, as the vibration is only produced by the healthy remaining vocal

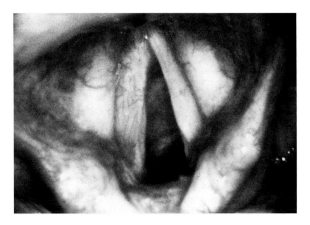

Fig. 1. Thick left pseudo vocal fold by scar formation after laser surgery.

cord. This disadvantage is in most cases more than compensated for by the fact that the remaining healthy vocal cord now has a counterpart with full mobility in the circoarytenoid articulation, thus in median position during phonation, resulting in a higher intensity of voicing and a longer phonation time (phonation quotient).

After *extended* laser cordectomy, the cicatric vocal fold is not always of sufficient thickness to produce a narrow glottic gap with phonation. Glottic phonation is in these cases practically absent, corresponding to an intense whispering. If the extension of the tumor and the providence of the surgeon leaves the ventricular folds intact, a phonation with the ventricular folds is achieved in most cases. The importance of ventricular fold phonation is often underestimated and in some cases ventricular fold resection is carried out, though not absolutely necessary. From the phoniatric point of view it has to be reminded that a ventricular fold phonation may have an often underestimated phonatory ability.

The data in table 1 are very informative concering the results of two different types of treatment, but they cannot give statistically significant results as tumor extension was different in both groups. The aim of a study comparing two surgical methods, should be the exact comparison of two groups with equal tumor extension and also an equal extension of resection. For a clinical follow-up study, it is only possible to fulfil these ideals partially. As for tumor extension, in both groups, we compared only those patients with stage T1a. Furthermore, we measured tumor extension and localisation according to preoperative drawings or intraoperative photos. In both groups *tumor exten-*

Table 2. Comparison of phonatory ability after treatment of T1a vocal fold carcinoma of 2 groups of equal extension

		Laser (n = 16)	p	Partial resection (n = 21)	Normal
Contentedness of patient with his voice					
Good		8		3	
Moderate		5		5	
Poor		3		13	
Psycho-acoustic evaluation of hoarseness					
Slight		5		2	
Moderate		6		10	
Extreme		5		9	
Phonation quotient, ml/s	$\bar{x}$	281	< 5%	502	140
	SD	70		227	
Frequency range of phonation, semitones	$\bar{x}$	22.4	< 1%	11.6	33
	SD	7.8		7.9	
Maximum intensity with crying, dB at 30 cm	$\bar{x}$	86.0	< 1%	77.6	> 90
	SD	8.8		5.9	
Computer analysis of voice purity by period autocorrelation, noise in % of total signal	$\bar{x}$	17.1	< 1%	65.5	0–8
	SD	8.9		31.2	

sion and *tumor localisation* are comparable and are nearly *equal*. The statistical analysis in table 2 refers to these two T1a vocal fold carcinoma groups of equal extension. (The extension of *resection* was not documented clearly enough for quantitative comparison.) In principle, it is never to be excluded that further factors are influencing the results: The two groups do not come from exactly the same time, but from two different, though overlapping, periods of time. The philosophy of treatment may have changed during this time and may have gone from eventual 'overtreatment' to eventual (at least suspected by extreme criticism) 'undertreatment', i.e. extension of resection may have been smaller with the 'laser group'. However, the statistically highly significantly different results should mainly be attributed to the two different surgical methods.

Prof. Dr. U. Reker, Phoniatry at the Department of Otorhinolaryngology, Head and Neck Surgery, University of Kiel, Arnold-Heller-Strasse 14, D–24105 Kiel (Germany)

Rudert H, Werner JA (eds): Lasers in Otorhinolaryngology, and in Head and Neck Surgery.
Adv Otorhinolaryngol. Basel, Karger, 1995, vol 49, pp 219–221

....

Endolaryngeal CO_2 Laser Microsurgery of Early Vocal Cord Cancer

A Retrospective Study

M. Csanády, J. Czigner, L. Sávay

ENT Department Albert Szent-Györgyi Medical School of Szeged
(Director: Prof. *J. Czigner*), Hungary

Endolaryngeal laser excision of early-stage vocal cord cancer is a discussed, but accepted procedure [1, 2]. This modality for the removal of vocal cord tumor has proved more effective than conservative surgery or radiotherapy [1, 3–6]. The indication must be established by an experienced oncologist [7–9]. The laser excision allows minimal invasive therapy at an early tumor stage (T1, T2), but has also been reported in laser therapy for T3 glottic cancer [9–12]. In the present study, 51 patients with early vocal cord cancer underwent CO_2 laser microsurgery and were followed up for 2–6.5 years.

Materials and Methods

A Storz laryngoscope was used for exploration and a Tungsram CO_2 laser set was applied at a power setting of 5–15 W in continuous mode and coupled to an Opton microscope combined with a micromanipulator. Laser excision was performed under general anesthesia. The vocal cord cancers were excised en bloc with an appropriate tumor-free margin. Fifty-one patients unterwent CO_2 laser cordectomy in the period May 1987 to December 1991. During the laser intervention frozen section histological control was performed to detect incomplete resection. The complications were very moderate. In 3 cases, bleeding from the paraglottic region occurred. One patient had subcutaneous emphysema and another had perichondritis. In 1 case, the protective cotton caught fire, but this was extinguished immediately. Some moderate postoperative edema was observed, but no tracheotomy was needed after the procedure. For the follow-up, we used an indirect laryngoscope, a laryngofiberoscope and biopsy in cases of a suspicion of tumor recurrence. The duration of hospitalization was on average 5 days. Complete healing took 5–6 weeks.

Table 1. Results after CO_2 laser cordectomy

	Tumor stage				
	T in situ	T1a	T1b	T2	total
Number of patients	7	32	9	3	51
Free of tumor after CO_2 laser excision					
n	7	28	6	2	43
%	*100*	*87*	*67*	*67*	*84*
Incomplete resection	–	1	–	–	1
Recurrence of tumor	–	3	3	1	7
Free of tumor after follow-up	7	30	9	3	49
Irradiation	–	3	1	–	4
Partial laryngectomy	–	1	2	1	4
Laryngectomy	–	1	–	–	1
Died of tumor	–	2	–	–	2
Died of unrelated disease	1	1	1	–	3

Results

Of the 51 vocal cord cancers excised by CO_2 laser, 7 were T in situ vocal cord cancer; after the CO_2 laser procedure, there was no evidence of recurrence. Twenty-eight of the 32 patients with T1a tumor had no recurrence after laser surgery. Four patients required additional therapy for recurrent tumor; laser resection was incomplete and 10 days later partial laryngectomy was performed. One patient required radiotherapy; the tumor recurred and total laryngectomy was then performed. All these patients are free of tumor. Two patients were irradiated after local tumor recurrence, but died later in consequence of the repeatedly recurring tumor or the developing metastases. There were 9 patients in the T1b subgroup. Six of them have been free from tumor recurrence since then. Three patients had recurrent tumor; 1 of them was irradiated (TeCo full course) after local recurrence, and 2 underwent partial laryngectomy. All of the patients in this subgroup are free of tumor. There were also 3 cases of stage T2 vocal cord tumor. In one patient, recurrence developed and partial laryngectomy was performed. All 3 patients have since remained free of tumor (table 1).

Discussion

The role of CO_2 laser excision of vocal cord cancer has increased recently, and our experience with laser microsurgery is likewise good. Surgery of vocal cord lesions requires skilled surgeons, selected patients and a well-defined indication. Endoscopic laser microsurgery is a preferred surgical intervention for the patient, because of the time factor and the many advantages of laser excision. However, there are difficulties during laser surgery particularly as regards excision in the anterior commissure and definition of the exact margins of the excised tumor. Clarification from this aspect requires the help of a pathologist to perform an intraoperative frozen section histological control. In the early stage of vocal cord cancers, our statistics revealed a success rate of 100% for T in situ, 87% for T1a, and 67% for T1b and T2 tumors, which demonstrates the efficacy of this surgical intervention. Including salvage surgery, the healing result was 94%. A comparison of the modalities of treatment of vocal cord cancer shows that the rate of recurrence is not higher than after conventional surgery or radiotherapy, and the voice quality is good in most cases.

References

1   Strong MS, Jakó GJ: Laser surgery in the larynx. Early clinical experience with continuous CO_2 laser. Ann Otol Rhinol Laryngol 1972;81:791–798.
2   Glanz H, Kimmlich T, Eichhorn T, Kleinsasser O: Behandlungsergebnisse bei 584 Kehlkopf-karzinomen an der Hals-Nasen-Ohrenklinik der Universität Marburg. HNO 1989;37:1–10.
3   Jakó GJ: Laser surgery of vocal cords. Laryngoscope 1972;82:2204–2209.
4   Davis RK, Jako GJ, Hyams VJ, Shapshay SM: The anatomical limitations of CO_2 laser chordectomy. Laryngoscope 1982;92:980–984.
5   Mendenhall WM, Parsons JT, Stringer SP, Cassisi NJ, Million RR: T1-T2 vocal cord carcinoma: A basis for comparing the results of radiotherapy and surgery. Head Neck Surg 1988;10:373–377.
6   Steiner W, Iro H, Petsch S, Sauerbrei W: Lasermikrochirurgische Behandlung von Larynxkarzinomen (pT2–4) Darstellung der Langzeitergebnisse; in Dühmke E, Steiner W, Reck R (eds): Funktionserhaltende Therapie des fortgeschrittenen Larynxzkarzinoms. Stuttgart, Thieme, 1991, pp 80–91.
7   Shapshay SM, Hybels RL, Bohigian RK: Laser excision of early vocal cord carcinoma: Indications, limitations and precautions. Ann Otol Rhinol Laryngol 1990;99:46–49.
8   Eckel HE, Thumfart WF: Laser surgery for the treatment of larynx carcinomas: Indications, techniques and preliminary results. Ann Otol Rhinol Laryngol 1992;101:113–118.
9   Thumfart WF: Early cancer of larynx. Lasersurgery of larynx-carcinomas: indications, techniques, follow up; Johnson JT, Didolkar MS (eds): Head and Neck Cancer. Amsterdam, Excerpta Medica Elsevier, 1993, vol 3, pp 215–222.
10 Steiner W, Aurbach G, Ambroch P: Minimally invasive therapy in otolaryngology and head and neck surgery. Minim Invas Ther 1991;1:57–70.
11 Motta G, Villari G, Motta G, Jr, Salerno G: The CO_2 laser in laryngeal microsurgery. Acta Otolaryngol (Stockh) 1986:(suppl 433).
12 Hirano M, Hirade Y: CO_2 laser for treating glottic carcinoma. Acta Otolaryngol 1988; (suppl 458): 154–157.

M. Csanády, MD, ENT Department, Albert Szent-Györgyi Medical School,
Tisza Lajos krt. 111, H–6725 Szeged (Hungary)

Rudert H, Werner JA (eds): Lasers in Otorhinolaryngology, and in Head and Neck Surgery.
Adv Otorhinolaryngol. Basel, Karger, 1995, vol 49, pp 222–226

....

Technique and Results of Transoral Laser Surgery for Small Vocal Cord Carcinomas

Heinrich Rudert

Department of Otorhinolaryngology, Head and Neck Surgery,
University of Kiel, Germany

Two hundred and forty-seven patients with laryngeal carcinomas have been treated by laser surgery at the Department of Otorhinolaryngology, Head and Neck Surgery, University of Kiel, between 1979 and 1992. In 114 Tis, T1a/b and T2 carcinomas laser surgery was the only form of the therapy.

Technique

All patients are operated under general anesthesia. The tracheal tube is protected by wet gauze. The larynx is exposed with a Kleinsasser laryngoscope which was modified by the addition of lateral suction channels [1]. The CO_2 laser is connected to an operation microscope with a 400-mm focus lens and a micromanipulator to guide the laser beam. Since the last 4 years, we have only used a Sharplan model. It generates a focus diameter of 0.25 mm at a working distance of 400 mm (4,000 W/cm^2 available with 2 W). Of two possible CO_2 laser applications, namely vaporization and excision, only the latter was used. Though vaporization is still described in the literature we feel it should not be used since it does not ensure complete tumor excision.

Excision in one piece, preferably as excisional biopsy, is used to remove small T1a carcinomas [2]. The tumor is grasped with small forceps containing a suction channel and then excised with a relatively small margin. The specimen is pinned on cork and examined in serial slides. The resulting tissue defect is as small as feasible, smaller than in conventional surgical excision and just large enough to ensure complete tumor removal. In carcinomas in situ and superficial T1a carcinomas, the muscular layer remains completely intact. In these cases the functional results are as good as after radiotherapy.

Larger tumors and tumors crossing the anterior primary commissure (T1b, T2) require a different technique of resection because they cannot be removed in one piece since the CO_2 laser beam can only be applied directly. The tumor has to be divided and removed in pieces [3, 4] (fig. 1). This opposes conventional oncological principles in surgery.

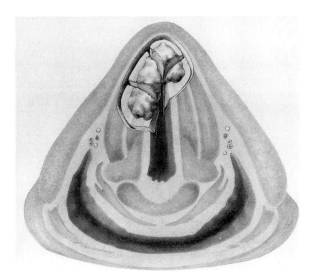

Fig. 1. Vocal cord carcinomas larger than T1a have to be divided into two or more parts. A hemostatic cut is achieved because of the cutting characteristics of the CO_2 laser.

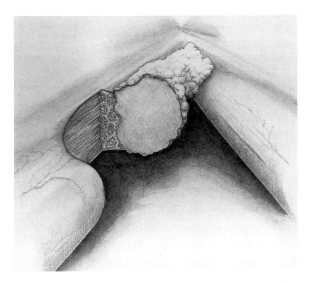

Fig. 2. The posterior part of the vocal cord carcinoma has been resected. The border-line between tumor and healthy tissue can be detected very well with the operating microscope. The residual tumor can be resected with a good margin of healthy tissue.

Table 1. Curative transoral laser surgery of glottic carcinomas (1979–1992)

Tumor classification	Pa-tients	No recur-rence	Recur-rence	Tumor related death
Tis	8	8	0	0
T1a	88	81	7	0
T1b	10	8	2	0
T2	8	7	1	0
Total	114	104	10	0

Average follow-up was 41 months.

It is only possible because of the characteristic CO_2 laser-tissue interaction. Using a modern micromanipulator with a small focus diameter of 0.25 mm and low laser power (1–2 W) tumor dissection is possible with almost immediate complete hemostasis. With the operating microscope, the borderline between tumor and muscle can be detected easily on the surface of the cut. The tumor is divided by a radial incision until healthy tissue is reached laterally (fig. 2). The separated parts can then be removed in sano. The ventricular fold can be removed if it hinders adequate exposure of the tumor. This technique was described by us in 1983 [5]. One disadvantage is that it prevents the development of a ventricular fold voice.

The operative specimens are reassembled and pinned together on cork. The deep resection margin is additionally marked. The pathologist can then prove (or disapprove) complete tumor excision by serial examination. Obviously, the tissue defect must be greater when larger tumors with tumor growth into the muscle are excised. The voice is, nevertheless, in most cases better than after open partial resection (frontolateral partial resection) with removal of all full compartment of the larynx [6].

The statistical evaluation of 114 Tis, T1 and T2 carcinomas treated in curative intention showed no recurrences among 8 Tis carcinomas (table 1). Out of 88 T1a carcinomas seven recurrences were observed, out of 10 T1b carcinomas and 1 out of 8 T2 carcinomas. No patient died related to tumor recurrence. Six recurrences were treated by repeated laser surgery or radiotherapy (fig. 3). Three patients had to undergo salvage laryngectomy. One patient refused further treatment.

In 7 of 10 patients recurrences were located in the anterior commissure (table 2). It is doubtless a problematic area. Histological studies revealed that in patients with highly differentiated carcinomas such as papillary or verrucous carcinomas and patients with multilocated highgraded dysplasias suffered tu-

Pat. nr.	age yrs	Tu-loc.	time to rec. months	loc. of rec.	therapy of rec.	rec. free months
		Recurrences of T1a - vocal cord carcinomas				
1	49	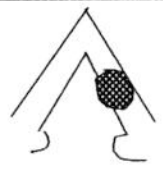	10	ant . comm.	irrad.	25
2	77	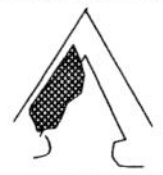	59	aryten.	laser	26
3	85	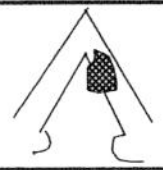	4	mid cord	laser	10
4	54	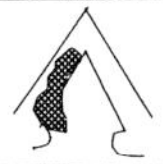	14	trans- glottic	laryngect. + ND	17
5	60	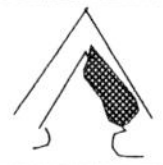	19	ant . comm.	laryngect.	70
6	43	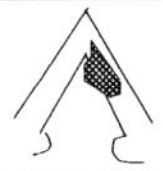	6	ant . comm.	irrad .	112
7	63	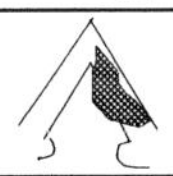	6	ant . comm.	refused	---
		Recurrences of T1b - vocal cord carcinomas				
8	73	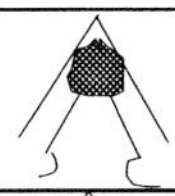	6	ant . comm.	irrad.	21
9	72	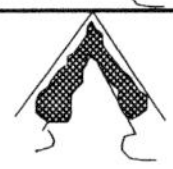	6	ant . comm.	laryngect.	21
		Recurrences of T2 - vocal cord carcinomas				
10	46	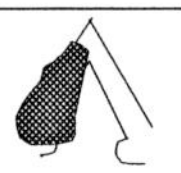	23	ant . comm.	laser	12

Fig. 3. Treatment of recurrent carcinomas.

mor recurrence more frequently. This also applies after treatment with radiotherapy or conventional surgery.

If histologic examination reveals that the tumor is not excised completely we either reexcise with the laser or in selected cases by conventional open partial resection.

Conclusion

Laser surgery of small vocal cord carcinomas (Tis, T1, T2) yields oncological results which are as good as after open vertical partial laryngectomy. The functional results are better after laser surgery and therefore we recommend it as the method of choice. The 5-year actuarial survival is at least equal but most likely better than after radiotherapy. The rate of recurrences is much higher after radiotherapy resulting in a higher rate of salvage laryngectomies. In 20% of the cases the tumor is completely removed by the initial biopsy [7] but the patients nevertheless undergo irradiation which is obviously overtreatment. Radiotherapy carries the risk of subsequent radiogenic carcinoma which is especially important in young patients. One also loses the option for radiotherapy of secondary malignancies increasingly developing in the head and neck area. We feel that the disadvantages of radiotherapy do not outweigh its only advantage which is a slightly better posttherapeutic voice when compared to laser surgery.

References

1   Rudert H: Instrumentarium für die CO_2-Laserchirurgie. HNO 1989;37:76–77.
2   Blakeslee D, Vaughan CW, Shapsay SM, Simpson GT, Strong MS: Excisional biopsy in the selective management of T_1-glottic cancer: A three-year follow-up-study. Laryngoscope 1984; 94:488–494.
3   Steiner W: Experiences in endoscopic laser surgery of malignant tumors of the upper aerodigestive tract. Adv Otorhinolaryngol. Basel, Karger, 1988, vol 39, pp 135–144.
4   Rudert H, Werner JA: Endoskopische Teilresektionen mit dem CO_2-Laser bei Larynxkarzinomen. I. Resektionstechniken. Laryngorhinootologie 1994;73:71–77.
5   Rudert H: Erfahrungen mit dem CO_2-Laser unter besonderer Berücksichtigung der Therapie von Stimmbandcarcinomen. Laryngorhinootologie 1983;62:493–498.
6   Reker U: Phonatory ability after surgery of vocal cord carcinoma of limited extention. A comparison between transoral laser microsurgery and frontolateral partial laryngeal resection. Adv Otorhinolaryngol. Basel, Karger, in press.
7   Stutsman AC, McGavran MH: Ultraconservative management of superficially invasive epidermoid carcinoma of the true vocal cord. Ann Otolrhinollaryngol 1971;80:507–512.

Prof. Dr. Heinrich Rudert, Department of Otorhinolaryngology, Head and Neck Surgery, University of Kiel, Arnold-Heller-Strasse 14, D–24105 Kiel (Germany)

Rudert H, Werner JA (eds): Lasers in Otorhinolaryngology, and in Head and Neck Surgery.
Adv Otorhinolaryngol. Basel, Karger, 1995, vol 49, pp 227–230

....

Technique and Results of Transoral Laser Surgery of Supraglottic Carcinomas

Heinrich Rudert

Department of Otorhinolaryngology, Head and Neck Surgery,
University of Kiel, Germany

Laser surgery for supraglottic carcinomas was discussed in the literature relatively late. It is less accepted than laser surgery for carcinomas of the vocal cord. Its advantages, however, are even more pronounced especially because of less postoperative morbidity when compared to conventional surgery.

The first publications regarding laser surgery for supraglottic lesions appeared in 1979 [1] and 1983 [2]. They also described the laser surgical treatment of few carcinomas of the epiglottis. Vertical splitting of the epiglottis for exposure of the supraglottic area was first described by Zeitels et al. [3]. They, however, did not split the tumors together with the epiglottis so that only small carcinomas were eligible for laser surgery if accessible for excisional biopsy. This may be the reason why supraglottic carcinomas are not yet included in the list of operative laser procedures. In Europe laser surgical excision of supraglottic carcinomas was started earlier [4–6].

At the University of Kiel, laser excision of supraglottic carcinomas have been performed since 1981, and, in the beginning, were done only sporadically. The laser has been used systematically since modern micromanipulators are available which generate a very small focus (0.25 mm in diameter). This allows to operate with low-power output (1–2 W) but high power density (2,000–4,000 W/cm^2) which in turn causes dissection in hemostasis. With the operating microscope one can also detect the borderline between tumor and healthy tissue on the cut surface and excise accordingly [7].

The operative procedures are usually carried out under general anesthesia. We use the bivalve laryngoscopes of Weerda or Steiner. For small tumors of the epiglottic border a laryngoscope as described by Lindholm may also be used. It is modified by adding suction channels. The upper blade of the bivalve laryngoscopes is placed in the vallecula and

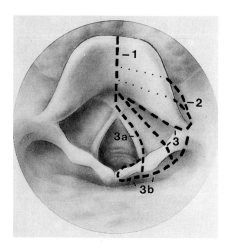

Fig. 1. Resection technique for advanced supraglottic carcinomas. The epiglottis is split in the midline vertically with the CO_2 laser (1). The second incision cuts along the vellecula or the tongue ground towards the plica pharyngoepiglottica (2). The third incision separates the aryepiglottic fold and meets the first incision (3). The third incision can include the ventricular fold (3a), the arytenoid and the medial wall of the piriform sinus (3b), depending on tumor localisation.

the base of the tongue. The lower blade is placed in the hypopharynx so that the tracheal tube is pushed dorsally towards the pharynx and larynx. Spreading of the instrument exposes the supraglottic area and the epiglottis.

Small carcinomas of the border of the epiglottis are excised in toto just like an excisional biopsy. If the tumor is larger and located centrally it is split vertically in the midline together with the epiglottis (fig. 1). The second incision cuts along the vallecula from the end of the first incision towards the plica pharyngo-epiglottica. The third incision starts at the aryepiglottic fold and meets the first incision and second incision anteriorly and distally to the tumor. The supraglottis can be resected in 2 pieces together with the tumor if all three cuts are connected. The second incision may also start laterally at the pharyngoepiglottic fold and be guided medially.

Splitting of the epiglottis also facilitates exposure and resection of tumors of the ventricular fold and the arytenoid region. It is superior to the direct endolaryngeal approach. Studies with cadaver specimens show that tumor growth in the preepiglottic fatty tissue is no contraindication for transoral laser surgery as long as tumor and healthy tissue can be differentiated with the operating microscope on the surface of the cut. Contraindications are tumors involving the infrahyoidal epiglottic (petiolus area) and tumors infiltrating the base of the tongue. The resection of one arytenoid cartilage is tolerable. However, routine tracheostomy is then recommended since we lost one of these patients due to aspiration pneumonia. Involvement of both arytenoids is a contraindication for this procedure since these patients always aspirate postoperatively.

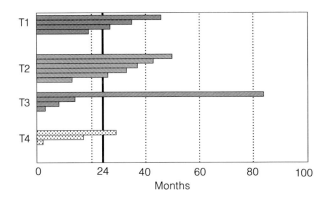

Fig. 2. Postoperative results after laser surgery of supraglottic carcinomas. Patients without recurrence.

Table 1. Curative transoral laser surgery of supraglottic carcinomas (1981–1993), early results (follow-up: average 24 months)

Tumor classifi- cation	Patients n	No recur- rence	Recur- rence	Died of secondary tumor	Tumor- unrelated death	Tumor- related death
T1	4	4	0	0	0	0
T2	11	7	1	1	2	1
T3	8	4	1	1	2	1
T4	7	3	2	0	2	1
Total	30	18	4	2	6	3

Forty-seven patients have been treated for supraglottic carcinomas with laser surgery between 1981 and 1993. In 17 patients the laser was only used for tumor debulking to avoid tracheostomy prior to subsequent laryngectomy to make the latter a clean and aseptic procedure. One also observed less recurrences around the tracheostoma.

Thirty patients were treated curatively (table 1). In 21 cases, additional radiotherapy was applied, 11 patients underwent neck dissection. Six patients died without evidence of tumor. Two patients died of a secondary malignancy without evidence of local disease. Three died of their primary tumor. Today, 18 patients are without evidence of local or metastatic tumor. Eleven of them with a minimum follow-up of 2 years (fig. 2).

The application of additional radiotherapy causes several problems. The development of edema makes the postoperative follow-up difficult, especially since recurrences have to be ruled out. The edema sometimes causes dysphagia and dyspnea which then have to be treated by laser surgical removal. Additional radiotherapy was therefore not applied in many cases. It is more preferable to perform elective supraomohyoidal neck dissection including levels II–IV and in some cases even V. The least extensive operation performed is a complete conservative neck dissection, if neck lymph nodes are manifest. Additional radiotherapy was applied to improve the prognosis in cases where the histology reveals involvement of more than one lymph node or extranodal disease.

Conclusion

Transoral supraglottic partial resection with the CO_2 laser is the operative method to treat supraglottic carcinomas with minimal morbidity for the patient. Tracheostomy is not required in most cases. Nutrition via gastric tube is in most cases only necessary during the first few postoperative days. There is practically no age limit. The oncological outcome is better than after radiotherapy and the functional results are distinctively better than after conventional surgery. We feel that transoral laser surgical resection is the future method of choice for the surgical treatment of most supraglottic carcinomas.

References

1   Vaughan CW: Transoral laryngeal surgery using the CO_2 laser: Laboratory experiments and clinical practice. Laryngoscope 1978;88:1399–1420.
2   Davis RK, Shapsay SM, Strong MS, Hyams VJ: Transoral partial supraglottic resection using the CO_2-laser. Laryngoscope 1983;93:429–432.
3   Zeitels SM, Vaughan ChW, Domanowski GF, Fullihan NS, Simpson GT II: Laser epiglottectomy: Endoscopic technique and indications. Otolaryngol Head Neck Surg 1990;103:337–343.
4   Steiner W: Experiences in endoscopic laser surgery of malignant tumors of the upper aerodigestive tract. Adv Otorhinolaryngol 1988;39:135–144.
5   Eckel HE, Thumfart WF: Vorläufige Ergebnisse der endolaryngealen Laserresektionen von Kehlkopfkarzinomen. HNO 1990;38:179–183.
6   Rudert H: Larynx- und Hypopharynxkarzinome. Endoskopische Chirurgie mit dem Laser: Möglichkeiten und Grenzen. Adv Otorhinolaryngol 1991(suppl I):3–18.
7   Rudert H, Werner JA: Endoskopische Teilresektionen mit dem CO_2-Laser bei Larynxkarzinomen. I. Resektionstechniken. Laryngorhinootologie 1994;73:71–77.

Prof. Dr. Heinrich Rudert, Department of Otorhinolaryngology, Head and Neck Surgery, University of Kiel, Arnold-Heller-Strasse 14, D–24105 Kiel (Germany)

Rudert H, Werner JA (eds): Lasers in Otorhinolaryngology, and in Head and Neck Surgery.
Adv Otorhinolaryngol. Basel, Karger, 1995, vol 49, pp 231–236

....

Management of Supraglottic Cancer: Selected Endoscopic Laser Resection and Postoperative Irradiation

R. Kim Davis[a], *John K. Hayes*[b]

Divisions of [a] Otolaryngology, Head and Neck Surgery, and [b] Radiation Oncology, University of Utah School of Medicine, Salt Lake City, Utah, USA

Endoscopic resection of T1 suprahyoid supraglottic cancers has been performed since the early 1980s [1]. Further, the ability to stabilize the airway without tracheotomy in selected advanced supraglottic cancer patients by performing CO_2 laser endoscopic subtotal supraglottic resections during the initial biopsy procedure has also been reported [2]. In these patients, complete epiglottectomy coupled in several instances with resection of the aryepiglottic folds and ventricular bands was accomplished without significant postoperative aspiration, hemorrhage, or subsequent airway obstruction. Safe postbiopsy extubations were possible in all these patients and tracheotomy was avoided.

In the ensuing 10 years since supraglottic resection with the CO_2 laser was first accomplished, the actual anatomical and functional limitations to such laser excision have been cautiously extended. This paper reviews the experience at the University of Utah Health Sciences Center with endoscopic supraglottic resection. The indications, contraindications, techniques of surgery, and results are presented.

Methods and Materials

A review of patients at the University of Utah School of Medicine who have undergone CO_2 laser resection of supraglottic cancer is presented. All patients with clinically apparent T1 or T2 supraglottic cancer first underwent preoperative CT scanning to determine the radiological presence or absence of pre-epiglottic space involvement by cancer. Patients with obvious pre-epiglottic space involvement were offered standard open laryngectomy, either supraglottic or total based on tumor extend. Selected patients who refused total laryngectomy, or who were not candidates for open supraglottic laryngectomy due to pulmonary limitations were treated endoscopically.

Supraglottic resections were accomplished in patients with airways secured by initial intubation with laser protected endotracheal tubes. Generally, newer metal endotracheal tubes were utilized with the cuffs of these tubes filled with saline. Moistened neurosurgical cottonoids were placed endoscopically through the glottis to further protect the cuffs of the endotracheal tubes from unintentional laser impact.

Supraglottic resection was accomplished by first positioning a bivalved laryngoscope with one blade in the vallecula, and the other blade pushing the endotracheal tube posteriorly. The epiglottis was divided vertically in the midline to an inferior extent approximately even with the level of the hyoid bone. This vertical incision was then joined by a horizontal incision extending from the pharyngoepiglottic fold medially to the vertical cut, allowing this portion of the epiglottis to be removed. In patients with primarily aryepiglottic fold cancers without tumor extension to the midline of the epiglottis, further resection was accomplished laterally and inferiorly, leaving the residual epiglottis intact. In all cases where the cancer approached the midline of the epiglottis the second half of the epiglottis was removed by bringing a horizontal incision from the contralateral pharyngoepiglottic fold to the previously placed midline incision.

With the epiglottis partially transected as described above, visualization of the upper aspect of the pre-epiglottic space was readily accomplished. Further resection was then carried out inferiorly in the pre-epiglottic fat anterior to the residual epiglottic cartilage. This incision line was joined to a vertical incision carried inferiorly through the epiglottic cartilage to the needed inferior extent. The lateral resection line was started by transecting the aryepiglottic fold at a craniocaudal level which allowed complete inferolateral resection of the tumor. This incision line could be placed as low as the body of the arytenoid cartilage if needed due to inferior tumor extension. When this resection line across the ary epiglottic fold was carried anteriorly, it was ultimately joined to the earlier-placed incision line in the pre-epiglottic space. Depending upon the inferior extent of the tumor, the false vocal cord was either included in this resection or not. As needed, resection was accomplished on one or both sides.

Once the tumor was grossly resected in this manner, further lines of laser excision either anteriorly in the pre-epiglottic space, infralaterally across the residual aryepiglottic fold or upper aspect of the soft tissue overlying the arytenoid cartilage, and anteriorly through residual false vocal cord were accomplished to gain the final margin of resection as guided by frozen section analysis. These secondary laser biopsies were appropriately oriented and sent for pathological review.

Hemostasis was provided by the laser and selected use of electrocautery where laser resection alone did not control bleeding. Typically, selective electrocautery was needed in the pre-epiglottic space, near the lateral extent of the pharyngoepiglottic fold, and in the upper aspect of the paraglottic space reached by transection of the aryepiglottic fold and ventricular band. After resection was completed, the patient was awakened and the endotracheal tube removed. Patients were carefully monitored in the recovery room. Intensive care monitoring was only necessary when other medical conditions required it.

Simultaneous neck dissection was accomplished in any patient with clinical or radiological evidence of metastatic spread to the neck. Modified radical neck dissection was accomplished on the side of nodal involvement. All patients received postoperative irradiation to the primary site and both necks, 50 Gy total in 1.8- to 2.0-Gy fractions. The primary tumor resection bed was boosted using shrinking fields to approximately 65 Gy.

Table 1. Subtotal supraglottic laryngectomy: University of Utah results – T2 or microscopic T3

Local control	23/24 = 96%
Survival	21/24 = 88%

All patients had postoperative irradiation and have been followed at least 4 years. There was only one local failure.

Table 2. Subtotal supraglottic laryngectomy: Morbidity Utah Series

Tracheotomy	0
Feeding tubes	3 (all T3 patients)
Hospitalization	2–4 days
Aspiration pneumonia	1/24

Feeding tubes were removed in 2 of 3 patients between 2 and 4 weeks postoperatively.

Results

Table 1 demonstrates the results with CO_2 laser supraglottic resection in 24 patients with supraglottic squamous cell cancer. Seventeen patients were staged clinically and by CT scanning to be T2 while 7 patients were T3 based on CT evidence of pre-epiglottic space involvement. These patients were followed for an average of 43 months with no patients lost to follow-up.

Local control rates in the T2 tumor group were 94% with laser excision and irradiation, and 100% when one salvage laryngectomy was included.

In the T3 group, local control was only 57% while ultimate local control including salvage laryngectomy was 86%. In the T3 group, survival was only 57% with death due to local failure in one, myocardinal infarction in one, and neck recurrence in the other patient.

Table 2 shows the morbidity seen in this series following subtotal supraglottic laryngectomy. As noted, no patient required tracheotomy. All patients requiring postoperative feeding tubes had T3 cancers and underwent full supraglottic laryngectomy. In 1 patient the feeding tube was needed only during radiation therapy, and subsequent to that.

Discussion

The initial results from CO_2 laser supraglottic resections at the University of Utah have previously been published [3]. All Utah patients have undergone supraglottic resection followed by postoperative irradiation with or without selected neck dissection based on the presence or absence of clinically apparent nodal disease at the time of the original staging. Postoperative irradiation was added to treat clinically inapparent microscopic disease at the primary site as well as to treat potentially present metastatic disease in the neck. As time has evolved and expertise with this technique increased, selected T1N0M0 and T2N0M0 patients are now undergoing supraglottic resection of the primary cancer coupled with bilateral functional neck dissections without postoperative irradiation.

Ultimate local control and survival rates are higher than in reported patients in the American literature who have undergone radiation therapy alone for stage II and III supraglottic cancers [4–6]. Although not rigorously studied, it is our impression that this approach has improved patient tolerance compared to open surgery or more aggressive radiation programs such as hyperfrationation. There are not at this time a sufficient number of patients treated by endoscopic resection to determine if this approach will provide cure rates as high as open partial supraglottic laryngectomy. Our results are similar, though, to the results seen at the University of Virginia where patients underwent conventional supraglottic laryngectomy and irradiation [7].

As noted earlier, the known treated T3 patients in this series either would have been excluded from open supraglottic laryngectomy due to poor pulmonary function, or refused total laryngectomy. These patients have been able to be treated endoscopically with minimal postoperative morbidity. None of these patients required tracheotomy. Of these 7 patients who underwent total supraglottic laryngectomy due to T3 cancer, 3 have needed feeding tubes with 1 patient ultimately needing a long-term gastrostomy tube. This patient had earlier suffered a stroke, had unilateral true vocal cord paralysis, and had refused total laryngectomy. No stage II patient required a postoperative feeding tube (table 2).

It is clear from this study that all grossly apparent cancer must be resected. Our data suggest that when all gross cancer is not removed, subsequent postoperative irradiation leads to a poor local control rate (57%). While patients who failed in this group were salvaged almost 70% of the time, such a low local control rate from the laser resection and postoperative irradiation is obviously unacceptable. Gross total resection, therefore, is important. Better success has been reported in this more advanced group of patients by Steiner [8]. His greater success almost certainly reflects the more extensive resections these patients have received. Specifically, Steiner has carried supraglottic resection extensively into the pre-epiglottic space and has even included the upper part of the thyroid ala where cancer spread has dictated this. Patients in his series with histologically positive surgical margins have been returned to surgery within days of the original procedure to further resect the cancer to obtain clear margins. This approach has probably allowed greater success with the more-advanced cancer patients.

Endoscopic resection has been safely accomplished in Utah and Germany in selected patients who are not candidates for open supraglottic laryngectomy. When all cancer is removed and postoperative irradiation is added, these patients have done very well. Endoscopic resection in all patients clearly confers less morbidity and is more cost effective than in patients treated with open supraglottic laryngectomy.

Endoscopic resection as described followed by postoperative irradiation has resulted in the local control rates which appear to be higher than control rates seen with conventional fractionation radiation therapy alone. This observation could only be proven by a subsequent study which would randomize patients between irradiation therapy alone and the approach described herein. Whether this approach would be better than newer radiation schemas with hyperfractionation, or versus simultaneous irradiation and chemotherapy is clearly not addressed. However, improved patient tolerance to therapy is expected compared to these more aggressive regimens. This also would need new studies, almost certainly multi-institutional, which may not be feasible un til the technology is better established.

When postoperative irradiation is added to any patient undergoing supraglottic laryngectomy, especially those treated by conventional techniques, morbidity clearly increases. As reflected in the data of Steiner [8], acceptable local control rates have been obtained in some of his patients without postoperative irradiation. This approach is being adopted in highly selected patients at the University of Utah as well. Clearly, all patients with any infrahyoid supraglottic cancer treated without postoperative irradiation also need to have treatment of the neck accomplished surgically. This is done by utilizing bilateral functional neck dissections.

References

1   Davis RK, Shapsay SM, Strong MS, Hyams VJ: Transoral partial supraglottic resection using the CO_2 laser. Laryngoscope 1983;93:429–432.
2   Davis RK, Shapsay SM, Vaughan CW, et al: Pretreatment airway management in obstructing carcinoma of the larynx. Otolaryngol Head Neck Surg 1981;89:209–214.
3   Davis RK, Kelly SM, Hayes J: Supraglottic resection with the CO_2 laser. Laryngoscope 1991;101:680–683.

4   Shimm DS, Coulthard SW: Radiation therapy for squamous cell carcinoma of the supraglottic larynx. Am J Clin Oncol 1989;12:17–23.
5   Robbins KT, Davidson W, Peters LJ, Goepfert H: Conservation surgery of T2 and T3 carcinomas of the supraglottic larynx. Arch Otolaryngol Head Neck Surg 1988;114:421–426.
6   Mendenhall WM, Parsons JT, Stringer SP, Cassisi NJ, Million RR: Carcinoma of the supraglottic larynx: A basis for comparing the results of radiotherapy and surgery. Head Neck 1990;12: 204–209.
7   Spaulding CA, Constable WC, Levine PA, Cantrell RW: Partial laryngectomy and radiotherapy for supraglottic cancer: A conservative approach. Ann Otol Rhinol Laryngol 1989;98: 125–129.
8   Steiner W: Results of curative laser microsurgery of laryngeal carcinoma. Am J Otolaryngol 1993;14:116–121.

R. Kim Davis, MD, Division of Otolaryngology, Head and Neck Surgery
University of Utah School of Medicine, 50 North Medical Drive, Room 3C120,
Salt Lake City, UT 84132 (USA)

Rudert H, Werner JA (eds): Lasers in Otorhinolaryngology, and in Head and Neck Surgery.
Adv Otorhinolaryngol. Basel, Karger, 1995, vol 49, pp 237–240

....

Functional Results following Partial Supraglottic Resection

Comparison of Conventional Surgery vs. Transoral Laser Microsurgery

Michael Köllisch, Jochen A. Werner, Burkard M. Lippert, Heinrich Rudert

Department of Otorhinolaryngology, Head and Neck Surgery,
University of Kiel, Germany

An external supraglottic partial resection or transoral laser surgery are two possible approaches in surgery for a limited supraglottic carcinoma. Besides the oncological results of these procedures the functional ones are extremely important for the patients. Based on the cases treated at the Kiel University, Department of Otorhinolaryngology, Head and Neck Surgery, these results will be discussed for both types of surgery.

The following aspects were considered when analyzing the two groups of patients, those treated by conventional surgery and those who underwent laser surgery: (1) placement and retention time of a nasogastric feeding tube as a criterion for postoperatively impaired swallowing; (2) placement of a tracheal stoma and duration of tracheotomy cannulation; (3) did supplementary therapeutic procedures contribute to impaired function?

Patients and Methods

A retrospective study includes 46 patients who had been treated by supraglottic partial resection for supraglottic carcinomas at the Kiel University Hospital of Otorhinolaryngology, Head and Neck Surgery. A conventional horizontal partial resection was performed in 20 cases (males, average age 63.1 ± 9.4 years) while a transoral supraglottic partial resection by CO_2 laser was done in 26 cases (7 females, 19 males, average age 62.4 ± 14.2 years). Regarding the extension of the tumors the two groups differed in that the group treated by conventional surgery (T1+2: 15 patients; T3+4: 5 patients) included some more small tumors than the group receiving treatment by laser (T1+2: 18 patients; T3+4: 8 patients).

Until 1975, Alonso's method was applied in conventional surgery (1960–1991). Following Mündnich and Banfai, a modified version of Alonso's technique has been used since 1976: a unilateral supraglottic partial resection was done, the skin flap was sutured to the remaining thyroid cartilage and the hyoid was resected. Laser surgery for partial supraglottic resections has been performed at the Kiel University Hospital since 1981. Rudert and Werner [1] published a precise description of the surgical procedure.

Results

Four of 26 patients were fed by nasogastric tube for more than 2 weeks after supraglottic resection by laser. In the group of patients who had undergone conventional surgery this measures had to be taken in at least 8 of the 20 patients. One must concede that the case histories had not been kept as accurately in the 1960s and 1970s as they were for the period when laser surgery was performed. In view of this fact, the number of patients provided with a gastric tube for more than 2 weeks probably was even higher in the group treated by conventional approach.

Five patients were tracheotomized in the laser group, a 6th patient had already been tracheotomized 49 years earlier because of diptheria with subsequent bilateral recurrent paresis of unknown cause. A tracheotomy was done in 17 of the 20 patients treated by conventional surgery. In 3 cases an extended epiglottidectomy was performed via lateral pharyngectomy so that a tracheotomy was not needed. Table 1 shows the period of time between placement and closure of the tracheostoma. A comparison between tracheotomized and non-tracheotomized patients of both groups indicates that laser surgery is superior from a functional perspective.

Eight of the 20 cases in the conventional group were diagnosed as having postoperative aspiration pneumonia, while this was the case in 3 of the 26 patients in the laser group. Of these 3 patients 1 was a female who developed aspiration pneumonia on the 4th day after surgery while the other 2 were males whose case histories are to be presented in the following since they were the only 2 cases in the group of 26 patients treated by laser surgery which were not satifactory from a functional point of view.

One of the cases was a 76-year-old male who had undergone laser surgery with a neck dissection for a T2N1M0 epiglottic carcinoma in 1990. The postoperative course was completely normal until the 4th week after surgery when radiation therapy started. Under radiation treatment the patient developed pronounced endolaryngeal edemas so that a tracheotomy had to be performed. Because of recurrent aspirations the nasogastric feeding tube had to be kept in place ut to the 30th postoperative week. Since the endolaryngeal edemas only subsided very slowly, the tracheostoma could be closed only after 130 weeks.

The second case was a 73-year-old male with a long laryngotracheal case history. In 1943, the patient had suffered from diphtheria and had been tracheotomized. A bilateral recurrent paresis of uncertain etiology developed during the following years. In 1970, an epiglottic carcinoma in the T2N1M0 stage was diagnosed and irradiated with 60 Gy. Laser surgery for a recidivation or possibly a radiogenous second carcinoma of the stage T2N1M0 was done in November 1992, resecting the left epiglottic half and the left fold. Due to the pre-existing bilateral recurrent paresis, the patient's ability to swallow without aspiration was extremely limited. The remaining larynx was removed for functional reasons in the 19th postoperative week at the patient's request. Because of recurrent aspirations the patient had been fed by nasogastric tube up to that point.

Discussion

The principles of the modern external supraglottic partial resection can be traced back to Alonso [2]. The functional results, which often are unsatisfactory, constitute a chief problem of this procedure. The postoperative morbidity rate after supraglottic partial resections is much higher than after simple laryngectomies [3]. Partial resection by laser surgery is an alternative to this conventional surgical procedure and has been employed more and more since the early 1980s [4–6].

The findings of the present study also indicate that better functional results can be achieved by laser surgery than by external partial resection of the larynx. Aspiration of saliva and food particles is the most common complication after supraglottic partial resection. The mortality rate because of aspiration pneumonia was stated to range from 27 to 40% and more [7, 8]. The present results also show a much lower rate of aspiration pneumonia for the laser group than for the group treated by conventional surgery. Because of the marked differences these results must be considered significant even though a retrospective comparative study will never achieve the significance of a prospective study.

An evaluation of the 2 cases in which laser surgery failed from a functional perspective points to the limitations of supraglottic partial resections by CO_2 laser. The success of this therapeutic method depends on an intact arytenoid region and on the limited extent of the resection in the retrolingual region. Postoperative radiotherapy can result in mucosal edemas causing serious functional problems with difficulties in swallowing – one should therefore be careful in prescribing such a therapy after laser surgery.

References

1   Rudert H, Werner JA: Endoskopische Teilresektionen mit dem CO_2-Laser bei Larynxkarzino-
    men. I. Resektionstechniken. Laryngorhinootologie 1994;73:71–77.
2   Alonso JM: Conservative surgery of cancer of the larynx. Trans Am Acad Ophthalmol Otola-
    ryngol 1947;51:633–642.
3   Kleinsasser O: Tumoren des Larynx und des Hypopharynx. Stuttgart, Thieme, 1987.
4   Davis RK, Shapsay SM, Strong MS, Hyams VJ: Transoral partial supraglottic resection using
    the CO_2 laser. Laryngoscope 1983;93:429–432.
5   Steiner W: Transoral microsurgical CO_2-laser resection of laryngeal carcinoma; in Wigand ME,
    Steiner W, Stell PM (eds): Functional Partial Laryngectomy. Berlin, Springer, 1984, pp 121–125.
6   Rudert H: Larynx- und Hypopharynxkarzinome – endoskopische Chirurgie mit dem Laser,
    Möglichkeiten und Grenzen. Arch Otorhinolaryngol 1991;(suppl I):3–18.
7   Leonard JR, Litton WB: Selection of the patient for conservative surgery of the larynx. Laryn-
    goscope 1971;81:232–252.
8   Siirala U, Pavolainen M: The problem of advanced supraglottic carcinoma. Laryngoscope
    1975;85:1633–1642.

Dr. Michael Köllisch, Department of Otorhinolaryngology, Head and Neck Surgery,
University of Kiel, Arnold-Heller-Strasse 14, D–24105 Kiel (Germany)

Rudert H, Werner JA (eds): Lasers in Otorhinolaryngology, and in Head and Neck Surgery.
Adv Otorhinolaryngol. Basel, Karger, 1995, vol 49, pp 241–244

Does External Access through Laryngofissure Widen the Indication for Laser-Surgical Partial Resection of the Larynx?

H.J. Neumann

Department of ENT Medicine, Regional Hospital of Halle, Germany

Endolaryngeal laser-surgical partial resection of the larynx offers a very differentiated choice of surgical procedures with a high degree of therapeutic efficiency [1]. However, the application of this technique in the treatment of laryngeal carcinomas may be restricted by a variety of factors. This restriction already starts with certain T2 tumors. In most cases of T3 tumors, a number of work teams decide against endolaryngeal laser-surgical partial resection, because the surgical intervention cannot be performed to the required extent owing to the individual biological and functional characteristics of the patient's disease [2–4]. The increased rate of recidivation or the continued growth of the tumor indicate that the compromise is not feasible in all cases. This compromise results from the limited technical possibilities of the use of laser beams, the narrowed field of vision at the distal end of the endoscope and the individual anatomical conditions. The objective of the operative treatment is the removal of the oncological disturbance under relevant mechanical and functional aspects, so that a lasting therapeutic success with minimum morbidity and appropriate aesthetic results can be achieved. Since the expanse of the tumor is given, the choice of the operative procedure is of vital importance.

Material and Methods

From 1992 to 1993, seven patients with T3 tumors of the larynx, in whom the exact expanse of the tumor could not be established endolaryngeally, underwent surgery from the outside through thyrectomy and laryngofissure, respectively. The individual operative steps are:

(1) Skin incision across the prominent part of the larynx up to the cricoid.
(2) Removal of a pre-thyroidal lymphatic node from the area of the cricothyreoid membrane.

(3) Thyrotomy or laryngofissure.
(4) Keeping the larynx open by inserting retractors.
(5) Demonstration of the expanse of the laryngeal tumor.
(6) Removal of the laryngeal tumor by means of a combined approach including conventional surgical techniques and laser-surgical possibilities.
(7) The site of the resection extends from the cricoid cartilage over the conic ligament on the interior surface of the thyroid cartilage up to the aryepiglottical plica. In the area of the posterior commissure the arytenoid cartilage – or the vocal process if necessary – is resected.

In this case, the resection proves to be technically a little more difficult than the endolaryngeal procedure.
(1) The resection of the anterior commissure is performed like a frontolateral partial resection.
(2) The operative procedure in all cases includes both halves of the larynx because of the expanse of the tumor.
(3) Placing a large-bore tracheal endoprosthesis according to Montgomery with the collaric shunt extending beyond the conic ligament.
(4) Placing a naso-esophageal nutrition probe postoperatively for 6–10 days.
(5) Layered closing of the wound, dressing.

Results

Since 1992, seven patients with T3 tumors and 1 patient with a T4 tumor of the larynx have been treated according to the described surgical concept in the ENT Department of the Regional Hospital of Halle. The follow-up treatment period was between 3 and 16 months. The T3 tumors proved to be carcinomas affecting one-half of the larynx from the supraglottis up to the subglottis and exceeding the anterior commissure to the opposite side. The vertical/lateral tumor expanse reached from the upper edge of the cricoid cartilage to below the aryepiglottic plica with deep infiltration of the paraglottic tissue structures. As a rule, the opposite side showed a smaller expanse of the tumor.

In the horizontal plane the anterior commissure and the cricothyroidal ligament were infiltrated in all cases.

The mucous membrane of the cricoid cartilage had in general to be resected down to a 10-mm-wide area.

The T4 tumor had spread bilaterally in the vertical plane infiltrating all three layers of the larynx and going beyond the aryepiglottic plica.

Five patients with T3 tumors were admitted for primary treatment. In 2 patients, laryngeal partial resection was performed because of an advanced T1b tumor or a T2 tumor with initial radiotherapy or else with endolaryngeal laser-surgical partial resection of the larynx.

So far, 1 T3 tumor patient has shown recidivation after 8 months in the sense of pT4N2M0 followed by laryngotomy, radical neck dissection and contralateral functional neck dissection. In the regular postoperative check-ups (every 6 weeks) under microlaryngoscopic conditions no further tumor recidivation has been observed up to now. Because of the very short period of assessment in the single case this finding should, however, be treated with caution. The average retention time for the tracheal endoprosthesis amounted to 6 weeks before decanulation.

Discussion

T3 tumors penetrate the fibroelastic structures of the larynx (elastic conus, thyreo-epiglottic ligament, vocal ligament, cricothyroid, Broyl's sinew) spreading in all directions of the paraglottic area.

An obvious alternative operative therapy is the partial resection of the larynx from the outside via thyrectomy or laryngofissure [5, 6]. Compared to the endolaryngeal techniques this approach has the following advantages:

(1) The objective of the operation is to make full use of the surgical possibilities in T3 tumors in order to diminish the number of laryngectomies. The surgical microscope allows for a very exact assessment of the laryngeal structures and the expanse of the tumor. The required extent of resection may be checked or corrected during the operation. The anatomic areas should be demonstrated at an optimum (anterior commissure, paraglottic space between cricoid cartilage and interior surface of thyroid cartilage, interior surface of cricoid cartilage, cricothyroid ligament, petiolus).

(2) A combination of the well-tried conventional partial resection of the larynx with the surgical possibilities provided by laser techniques extends the range of surgery. By using laser almost all anatomic areas can be reached.

(3) Also, in the case of tumor recidivation after endolaryngeal partial resection surgical intervention via thyrotomy may offer a last chance to avoid laryngectomy.

(4) Controlling hemorrhage is without any problems.

The indications for surgical and/or radiotherapeutic treatment of the regional lymphatic node compartment remain the same. The described surgical concept is restricted by the following facts:

(1) The surgical requirements are higher than those for the endolaryngeal procedures. Postoperative hospital treatment as well as out-patient treatment is considerably longer. The discomfort for the patient is increased.

(2) The retention time for the tracheal endoprosthesis according to Montgomery differs widely, mainly depending on the intralaryngeal repair process.

As a rule, breathing is reliably ensured through the large-bore endoprosthesis. The most frequent breathing disturbances are caused by: (a) laryngostenoses during the healing process; (b) long-lasting edema of the arytenoid cartilage; (c) instable projecting epiglottis, and (d) by long-standing inflammations with more difficult decanulation.

(3) As a rule, after the operation a nasoesophageal nutritional probe is required for 5–10 days.

(4) The quality of the voice regarding communication may be looked upon as satisfactory. If the larynx heals in a tube shape, this results in a strongly muffled voice with diminished sound retention time.

Postoperative check-ups should be done at intervals of 4–6 weeks using microlaryngoscopy, since the oncological condition can be ascertained only histologically due to often long-lasting granulation processes. If necessary, the check-up has to be combined with an endolaryngeal laser-surgical treatment in order to keep the breathing tract free. When a new tumor is detected laryngectomy almost invariably appears to be the only feasible therapeutic consequence. The increase in the range of surgical possibilities for laryngeal partial resections through the combination of conventional surgical procedures (frontolateral partial resection according to Lerouxrobert, hemilaryngectomies according to Hautant) and the techniques of laser surgery should be considered as a possible alternative if the required extent of the surgical intervention cannot be achieved with the endolaryngeal laser-surgical procedure.

The postoperative results obtained so far by means of the described surgical procedure give rise to cautious optimism concerning the avoidance of laryngectomies.

References

1   Steiner W: Laserchirurgie im HNO-Bereich (Laserchirurgie zur Behandlung maligner Tumoren des oberen Aerodigestivtraktes). Arch Otorhinolaryngol 1987;(suppl 2):8–18.
2   Eckel HE: Topographische und klinisch-onkologische Analyse lokoregionärer Rezidive nach transoraler Laserchirurgie zur Behandlung von Kehlkopfkarzinomen. Laryngorhinootologie 1993;72:406–411.
3   Rudert H: Larynx- und Hypopharynxkarzinome – Endoskopische Chirurgie mit dem Laser: Möglichkeiten und Grenzen. Arch Otorhinolaryngol 1991;(suppl 1):3–18.
4   Thumfart WF, Eckel HE: Endolaryngeale Laserchirurgie zur Behandlung von Kehlkopfkarzinomen. Das aktuelle Kölner Konzept. HNO 1990;38:174–178.
5   Kleinsasser O: Tumoren des Larynx und des Hypopharynx. Stuttgart, Thieme, 1987, pp 169–185.
6   Neel H III: Laryngofissur mit Chordektomie und vertikale Kehlkopfresektion. Arch Otorhinolaryngologie 1991;(suppl 1):19–21.

Priv.-Doz. Dr. med. H.J. Neumann, HNO-Klinik des Bezirkskrankenhauses Halle,
Röntgenstrasse 12, D–06120 Halle (Germany)

Rudert H, Werner JA (eds): Lasers in Otorhinolaryngology, and in Head and Neck Surgery.
Adv Otorhinolaryngol. Basel, Karger, 1995, vol 49, pp 245–249

....

Analysis of Recurrences after Transoral Laser Resection of Larynx Carcinomas

Walter Franz Thumfart [a], *Hans Edmund Eckel* [b], *Georg Mathias Sprinzl* [a]

[a] Universitäts-Hals-Nasen-Ohrenklinik Innsbruck
  (Vorstand: Universitätsprof. *W.F. Thumfart*), Innsbruck, Österreich;
[b] Universitäts-Hals-Nasen-Ohrenklinik Köln
  (Direktor: Universitätsprof. *E. Stennert*), Köln, Deutschland

A transoral laser-assisted surgical method has been developed based upon the microlaryngoscopic pathway developed by Kleinsasser [1], enabling the curative treatment of Tis, T1 and T2 carcinomas primarily of the glottis but also the subglottis and supraglottis. Before Strong and Jako's [2] 1972 introduction of the CO_2 laser in the endolaryngeal microsurgery the only indication given for the excision of laryngeal carcinomas was in cases involving microcarcinomas of the ligamentary glottis showing only limited expanse and no impedement of vocal cord movement. In cases involving bilateral vocal cord carcinomas (T1b) an indication was only given in isolated incidences. In these cases a bilateral resection was generally advisable [1, 3]. Information regarding the microlaryngoscopic resection of subglottic and supraglottic carcinomas prior to the introduction of laser surgery could not be found in the recent literature.

Material and Methods

From 1986 to 1992 at the University Ear, Nose and Throat Clinic in Cologne, 204 patients experienced transoral surgical procedures in the curative therapy of laryngeal carcinomas including 169 glottis, 28 supraglottis and 7 subglottis tumors [4]. Oncologically, 18 cases involved carcinoma in situ, 179 cases demonstrated infiltrating growth of platelet epithelium carcinomas, 6 of the tumors were verrucous and 1 tumor was an adenocarcinoma. Among the 169 glottis tumors, 42 had reached the anterior vocal chord commissure or the contralateral vocal cord. Twelve further carcinomas were isolated in the region of the anterior commissura. Thirty-nine carcinomas had reached the mucosa above the processus vocalis of the arytenoid cartilage dorsally. Among the 28 supraglottic tumors, 11

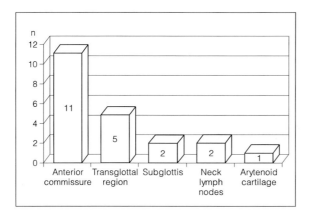

Fig. 1. Localization of 21 recurrences after transoral laser partial laryngectomies.

were located in the vestibular fold, 14 in the laryngeal epiglottis region or in the aryepiglottic fold, 2 in the region of the arytenoid cartilage, and 1 in the petiolus region of the epiglottis.

Results

To date (follow-up of 12 months to 7 years, mean of 37 months, 143 patients over 2 years) 21 locoregional recidivations were discovered among the patients treated by this method. Among these, 16 tumors were located in the larynx, 2 were isolated in the lymph nodes of the neck and 3 in the larynx and lymph nodes of the neck simultaneously.

Of the 19 larynx recidivations 10 were located alone in the region of the anterior commissure (fig. 1) and 5 in the so-called transglottic region. The treatment of 14 of these patients consisted of a laryngectomy (including a neck dissection where necessary). Two further patients were subjected anew to transoral laser resections, one of which was a supraglottic partial larynx resection according to Alonso, and the other a subtotal laryngectomy with an epiglottis interposition according to Tucker and two neck dissections without any further larynx treatments. Metastases located distant from the primary tumor were only found among primary tumors which could not be kept in check. To date, 5 patients have died due to tumor recidivations (fig. 2). One of these was a patient who after the discovery of a most probably surgically curable recidivation refused all treatment and shortly thereafter committed suicide. According to the observations to date, recidivations were found after resections of subglottic and supraglottic carcinomas more commonly than among glottic tu-

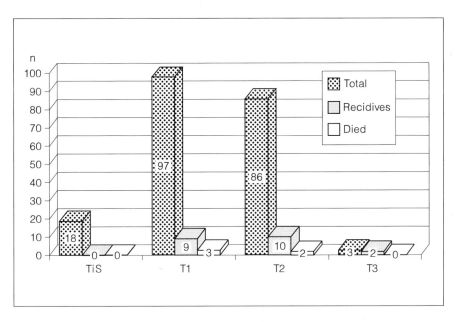

Fig. 2. Ratio of recurrences in relation to the size of cancer.

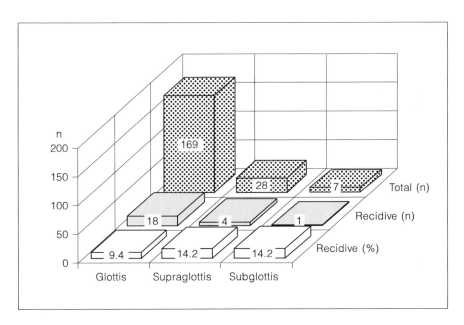

Fig. 3. Recurrences after transoral laser resection of glottic, subglottic and supraglottic carcinomas (n = 204).

mors (fig. 3). Approximately 70% of all recidivations observed manifested within the first year after the conclusion of the primary treatment, and over 80% manifested within the first 2 years.

Discussion

As was expected, local and regional recidivations were found more often following treatment of subglottic or supraglottic carcinomas; this observation correlates to the well-known worse prognosis of carcinomas in this region as compared to glottic carcinomas [5]. The low number of isolated lymph node metastases is probably due to the routinely performed prophylactic (mostly bilateral) neck dissection for the sanitation of the lymph passages among subglottic and supraglottic carcinomas. The chronological occurrence of recidivations – though not yet completely evaluable due to the relatively short follow-up period of a portion of the patients – appears to be comparable to the results following the conventional surgical therapy of laryngeal carcinomas [3]: The majority of the recidivations manifested in the first 2 years after conclusion of the therapy. In this time period, the follow-up treatment must be especially intense. Control microlaryngoscopic examinations after 6 and 12 weeks have proven invaluable in the Cologne clinic for the early assessment of residual tumors. Ambulatory low magnification laryngoscopic control examinations have occurred every 3 months. This time period is most probably too long, as recidivations are thus often diagnosed after they have reached a stage requiring a total laryngectomy in order to stop the tumor proliferation.

The topographical analysis of the recidivations has shown that the absolute majority of the recidivations occurred in the region of the anterior vocal chord commissure (11 of 21 locoregional recidivations). Among the 21 recidivations observed among the 204 endolaryngeally operated patients, 2 were found isolated in the region of the lymph nodes of the neck and 19 in the larynx. Among the 19 patients who later showed recidivations in the larynx, 16 had originally suffered glottis carcinomas and 3 supraglottic tumors. The 11 recidivations in the region of the anterior commissure were diagnosed amongst 4 of the 12 (33%) patients who had originally suffered carcinomas of the anterior commissure, 4 of the 42 (10%) patients with vocal chord carcinomas reaching the anterior commissure, 2 patients with vocal chord carcinomas which originally did not appear to reach the anterior commissure and 1 patient with a petiolus carcinoma. This means that of 16 local recidivations which were observed among 179 patients after endolaryngeal resection of carcinomas of the glottis, 10 (63%) were located in the region of the anterior commissure.

References

1 Glanz H, Kimmich T, Eichhorn T, Kleinsasser O: Behandlungsergebnisse bei 584 Kehlkopfkarzinomen an der Hals-Nasen-Ohrenklinik der Universität Marburg. HNO 1989;37:1–10.
2 Strong MS, Jako GJ: Laser surgery in the larynx. Early clinical experiences with continuous CO_2 laser. Ann Otol 1972;81:791–798.
3 Kirchner A, Owen JR: Five hundred cancers of the larynx and the pyriform sinus. Results of treatment by radiation and surgery. Laryngoscope 1977;87:1288–1303.
4 Eckel HE: Topographische und klinisch-onkologische Analyse lokoregionärer Rezidive nach transoraler Laserchirurgie zur Behandlung von Kehlkopfkarzinomen. Laryngo Rhino Otol 1993;72:406–611.
5 Kleinsasser O: Mikrolaryngoskopie und endolaryngeale Mikrochirurgie, ed 3. Stuttgart, Schattauer, 1991.

Univ.-Prof. Dr. med. Walter Franz Thumfart, Universitäts-Hals-Nasen-Ohrenklinik,
Anichstrasse 35, A–6020 Innsbruck (Austria)

Rudert H, Werner JA (eds): Lasers in Otorhinolaryngology, and in Head and Neck Surgery.
Adv Otorhinolaryngol. Basel, Karger, 1995, vol 49, pp 250–253

....

Transoral Laser Surgery of Laryngeal Carcinomas

State of the Art in Sweden

C.-E. Lindholm[a], *Å. Elner*[b]

Departments of Oto-Rhino-Laryngology,
[a] Örebro Medical Center Hospital, and [b] University Hospital, Lund, Sweden

In 1986, leading Swedish otolaryngologists and oncologists with special interest in laryngeal cancer agreed on recommendations given in a treatment scheme against this disease.

The recommendations stated that all laryngeal glottic and supraglottic cancers classified as Tis to T3 (UICC 1985) should be treated by primary radiotherapy with curative intent. T4 cases should be treated more individually by laryngectomy with pre- or postoperative irradiation and all stages of subglottic cancers should be treated according to decisions made by the responsible physician. It may seem rather radical to launch such recommendations but they should be seen in the light of the high standard of both diagnostic and therapeutic radiology in Sweden since the time when Konrad Roentgen in Uppsala discovered the medial use of X-rays in 1895.

Material and Methods

The recommended irradiation for Tis and T1a tumors have generally been followed in Sweden. However, in Lund (ÅE) and partly in Uppsala-Örebro (CEL) laser surgery has been used as an alternative therapy in these tumors. An inquiry to the larger hospitals in Sweden revealed that approximately 150 cases of Tis and T1a cancers have been treated with CO_2 laser surgery in Sweden, some as a salvage procedure after failed irradiation therapy. Eighty cases have been treated by CO_2 laser in Lund and Uppsala-Örebro and are presented in table 1.

The treatment of Tis tumors consisted of CO_2 laser evaporation down to the vocalis muscle and in some cases also involving part of the muscle. The T1a tumors were treated

Table 1. Cases

	ÅE		CEL		Total
	M	F	M	F	
Tis	20	4	9	0	33
T1a	32	2	12	1	47
Total	52	6	21	1	80

ÅE = Patients from Lund; CEL = patients from Uppsala-Örebro.

by CO_2 laser excision of the entire vocal fold from the vocal process to the anterior commissure (in the CEL series, a few reached the anterior commissure therefore the anterior commissure a part of the opposite vocal fold was also removed). All patients were followed up more than 1 year. The combined results of the two series are given as there was no significant difference in the achieved results.

Results

Among the 33 patients with glottic Tis tumors 8 developed recurrent disease (about 25%). These patients had an interval of 4–60 months to tumor recurrence.

All recurrent Tis tumors received a secondary CO_2 laser treatment and 5 of them healed. Three tumors recurred a second time. Two of these were cured by an additional CO_2 laser treatment and the third one, which had become an invasive carcinoma, received radiotherapy and healed.

Four of 47 patients with T1a vocal fold cancer developed recurrent disease (about 9%). Two of these patients were considered to have recurrent invasive T1a tumor and received radiotherapy and have since been tumor free.

The two remaining recurrences were classified as Tis and were treated with the CO_2 laser. One of these patients has remained tumor free but the second has developed cancer in situ and pathology described as squamous cell papilloma on both vocal cords repeatedly and there is some doubt regarding the nature of the recurrences.

The interval to recurrent T1a tumor was for 3 patients 48, 42 and 20 months, respectively, and for the remaining patient with recurrent disease five times the first recurrence occurred within 6 months.

Discussion

Already at the time when the therapy scheme was agreed upon there was some controversy as how to treat glottic Tis, small glottic T1a tumors and glottic T3 tumors. Radiotherapy of Tis and T1a tumors could be considered an 'overkill' and the T3 tumors could, according to a literature report [1], be cured in only approximately 50%. The rest had to have salvage laryngectomy once persistent disease was discovered.

Laser surgery was, already at the time of agreement to the treatment, reported to cure small vocal fold cancers in as high a percentage as did irradiation [2]. The drawback was in general slightly changed voice which has been verified by the Lund group [3]. The most striking result in the present series, however, was the 25% recurrence rate in glottic in situ carcinomas. One reason for this outcome may be a persistent 'unrest' in the epithelium leading to a new pathology, which could be classified as Tis. Another explanation may be the doubtful surgical margin due to the contradictory aim of function and preservation. However, all Tis lesions ultimately have been controlled so far.

The 9% recurrence rate in the glottic T1a carcinomas following laser surgery was comparable with other similar series [4–6] and with the results after radiotherapy [7]. Laser surgery is very cost effective with in general 3 days' hospitalization compared with up to 6 weeks' treatment by radiotherapy even if the latter may be given as an out-patient procedure in most instances.

Regarding T3 tumors there is to our knowledge still no follow-up presented in Sweden regarding the outcome of primary radiotherapy. Our personal experience is that it is difficult to get valid information in the postirradiation period whether there is persistent tumor or not. Radiographic methods and direct microlaryngoscopy with multiple biopsies are often inconclusive in these cases at the beginning. At least 3–4 months may elapse before the true nature of the therapy result is encountered. During this delay, there may be obvious chances of tumor spread. Until proper follow-up results are presented there is some doubt whether this mode of therapy is the method of choice in view of survival rate.

References

1   Harwood AR, Hawkins NV, Beale FA, Rider WD, Bryce DP: Management of advanced glottic cancer. A ten-year review of the Toronto experience. Int J Radiol Oncol Biol Phys 1979;5:473–476.
2   Blakeslee D, Vaughan CW, Simpson GT, Sharpshay SM, Strong SM: Excisional biopsy in the selective management of T1 glottic cancer: A three-year follow-up study. Laryngoscope 1984; 94:488–494.
3   Elner Å, Fex S: Carbondioxide laser as primary treatment of glottic Tis and T1a tumors. Acta Otolaryngol (Stockh) 1988;449:135–139.

4   Olsen KD, Thomas JV, Desanto LW, Suman VJ: Indications and results of cordectomy for early glottic carcinoma. Otolaryngol Head Neck Surg 1993;108:277–282.
5   Steiner W: Results of curative laser microsurgery of laryngeal carcinomas. Am J Otolaryngol 1992;14:116–121.
6   Rudert H: Larynx- und Hypopharynxkarzinome: Endoskopische Chirurgie mit dem Laser – Möglichkeiten und Grenzen. Erläuterungen zum vorliegenden Referat. Arch Otorhinolaryngol 1991;(suppl 1991/II):14–18.
7   Fernberg J-O, Ringborg U, Silfversvärd C, Ewert G, Haglund S, Schiratzki H, Strander H: Radiation therapy in early glottic cancer. Acta Otolaryngol (Stockh) 1989;108:478–481.

Carl-Eric Lindholm, MD, PhD, Department of Otorhinolaryngology,
Örebro Medical Center Hospital, S–70185 Örebro (Sweden)

Rudert H, Werner JA (eds): Lasers in Otorhinolaryngology, and in Head and Neck Surgery.
Adv Otorhinolaryngol. Basel, Karger, 1995, vol 49, pp 254–258

....
Transoral Laser Surgery for Glottic Cancer

R. Kim Davis

Division of Otolaryngology, Head and Neck Surgery, John A. Dixon Laser Institute,
University of Utah School of Medicine, Salt Lake City, Utah, USA

Transoral CO_2 laser excision of carcinoma in situ and early T1 glottic cancer was introduced in America by Vaughan et al. [1] in the 1970s. At this time,
it was felt that resection of the arytenoid cartilage coupled with resection of
the soft tissue of the true vocal chord was absolutely contraindicated due to
the high likelihood of postoperative aspiration. There was also significant concern that when cancer extended to the body of the arytenoid, paraglottic extension of cancer beyond the safe limits of laser cordectomy would often be
present, thereby contraindicating endoscopic resection. With this premise as a
guiding principle, the anatomical limitations to resection of glottic cancer were
investigated by Davis et al. [2]. In a cadaver study, cancer excision could be accomplished at a right angle across the vocal process of the arytenoid through
the paraglottic space to the thyroid cartilage. This was determined to be the
posterolateral extent to which safe laser excision could be accomplished. Anteriorly, it was determined that the anterior commissure tendon (Boyle's ligament) could be easily approached and resected. The anterior inferior limitation to resection was felt to be the cricothyroid membrane through which
tumor would escape to the soft tissues of the neck, thereby contraindicating
any conservation operation. These limitations to transoral CO_2 laser resection
of glottic cancer have largely remained in place in America ever since that
time.

The most significant American paper reporting results of transoral CO_2
laser excision on T1 glottic cancer came from Boston University [3]. Patients
underwent excisional biopsy of T1 glottic cancer at the time of their definitive
staging endoscopy. All cancers were excised versus vaporized. Once the main
tumor specimen had been excised it was appropriately oriented and sent for a

histopathological review. Additionally, standard microsurgical biopsies were taken in several areas of the excisional bed to prove the presence or absence of cancer extension into the underlying vocalis muscle. Where final margins were found to be free of cancer after excisional biopsy, and where the deeper biopsies in vocalis muscle revealed no cancer, patients were determined to have had a complete cancer excision, and received no further treatment. On the other hand, where resection margins or deep biopsies were positive for cancer, then the patients were offered either open vertical partial laryngectomy or, more typically, full-course radiation therapy.

In the Boston University study, 50 patients underwent laser excision alone and had a three year NED rate of 92%. In 34 patients where cancer was found in the biopsies taken in vocalis muscle after laser excision, radiation therapy was given resulting in a 3-year NED rate of 85%. All 4 patients with extensive cancer who underwent vertical partial laryngectomy obtained 100% control at 3 years. For the total group, 90% of patients had local control by the above-mentioned methods. It is important to note in this study that reported local control was obtained from the primary therapies, and did not include salvage surgery.

A similar study was undertaken at the University of Utah where 70 patients were selected for laser excision or definitive irradiation therapy. Patients with T1a carcinoma of the true vocal cord underwent laser excision according to the Boston regimen. None of these patients had positive margins, and the 5-year NED rate was 93% [4]. Patients with stage T1b received radiation therapy with only 67% rendered free of cancer by radiation alone. Several other papers in the American literature report results of laser excision ranging from 3-year NED rates of 80–92% [5, 6].

Stage II glottic cancer (T2N0M0) has generally been treated in America utilizing radiation therapy. The alternative to this has been open vertical partial laryngectomy. The current status or definitive radiation therapy is reflected in several papers.

At the University of Virginia the 3-year disease-free survival for irradiated patients with stage II glottic cancer was 75.5% [7]. Failure was most commonly seen in patients with persistent hoarseness after radiotherapy and in patients with impaired true vocal cord mobility before cancer therapy. In a large series from the MD Anderson Hospital of 114 patients with stage II glottic cancer, the recurrence rate following definitive radiotherapy was 32% [8]. In a series from the Geisinger Medical Center 48 patients with T2 glottic cancer underwent definitive irradiation [9]. Local control at 3 years was obtained in 73%. Patients with impaired vocal cord mobility or anterior commissure cancer were identified as being at increased risk of recurrence after primary radiation therapy.

A review of the world literature for T2 glottic cancer shows similar control rates for T2 cancer treated by irradiation alone, specifically 60–70%. In a paper from Lille, France, 24 patients underwent primary radiotherapy for T2 lesions [10]. Thirty percent of patients with extension to the anterior commissure, and 5 of 6 patients with tumor extension to the arytenoid cartilage failed primary irradiation. Clearly, in both the American and world literature, radiotherapy has a higher probability of failure to control these cancers with either anterior commissure extension or, more specifically, extension of tumor to the area of the arytenoid cartilage.

In light of the problems with radiotherapy in T2 cancers with extension of disease either to the anterior commissure or to the arytenoid cartilage area, the vast majority of American head and neck surgeons would favor conventional open vertical partial laryngectomy in these patients. In the reported American literature, all series with the exception of this paper, have used only open techniques.

Steiner [11], in Göttingen, Germany, has reported excellent results in stage II glottic cancer patients utilizing transoral CO_2 laser microsurgery for these lesions. His approach has shown that the traditionally accepted limitations to transoral glottic cancer surgery earlier discussed were in fact too conservative. In light of Steiner's excellent results, and in light of the poor success with more extensive T2 glottic cancer treated by conventional radiation alone, a prospective nonrandomized study of patients with T2b glottic cancers was undertaken at the University of Utah.

Patients with stage II glottic cancer with impaired true vocal cord mobility were taken to microlaryngoscopy. Patients were excluded from analysis if the true vocal cord could not be fully visualized endoscopically from the anterior commissure through and including the arytenoid area. Patients were intubated with laser-protected tubes with moistened neurosurgical cottonoids placed through the glottis to protect the underlying cuffs of these endotracheal tubes. Laser excision was started posteriorly immediately in front of the vocal process of the arytenoid by cutting tangentially across the tumor toward the lateral paraglottic space and thyroid cartilage. Cutting vertically through tumor in this manner (as described by Steiner) allowed the depth of tumor extension to be determined. Once this was accomplished, cancer was excised posteriorly in the area of the arytenoid cartilage. In all cases, the vocal process of the arytenoid was fully transected and excision was carried out immediately adjacent the arytenoid body. Cancer present posterolateral to the body of the arytenoid and in the upper portion of the arytenoid body was also excised. If cancer extended posterior to the arytenoid, the full arytenoid cartilage itself was excised.

Cancer invasion was not seen directly in the arytenoid cartilage, but at least subtotal removal of the arytenoid was necessary in most patients to ensure complete excision of the posterior tumor.

Once the posterior aspect of the tumor was resected, the anterior aspect of cancer was excised in either one or two specimens based on the full anterior extent of tumor. Where tumor extended to the anterior commissure, the anterior commissure was fully exposed, and in all cases the anterior perichondrium was fully excised. In this Utah series, all patients underwent postoperative irradiation.

Local control rate at 2 years was 92% (11 of 12 patients). The 1 patient who developed local failure was salvaged by total laryngectomy, yielding an ultimate local control rate of 100%. None of these patients required tracheotomy, and 2 of 12, or 17%, required postoperative feeding tubes for 2–4 weeks. Importantly, both patients requiring feeding tubes had very extensive cancers where an extended vertical partial laryngectomy had been accomplished to include the previously mentioned complete excision of the true cord, the arytenoid cartilage, vocal cord, aryepiglottic fold, and hemiepiglottis at the site of the lesion.

While the Utah series was indeed limited, it did show a local control rate of 92% in T2b glottic cancer patients. Obviously, no statistically valid statement can be made about such a small group. All Utah patients were given postoperative irradiation which could in fact reflect overtreatment of these patients. Clearly, the results obtained by Steiner [11] would suggest that postoperative irradiation is not necessary in all T2b patients. On the other hand, if a more extensive series would show local control rates of greater than 90% in these patients, it can be stated that this degree of local control is higher than control rates reported in the world literature with radiation alone for T2b glottic cancer.

In light of this investigation and in light of the results reported by Steiner, it certainly appears oncologically sound to transorally excise T2 glottic cancer. Obviously, it is critical that adequate visualization be obtained in these patients, and it is further critical that adequate cancer excision be accomplished. This necessarily will include skeletonization of the arytenoid cartilage with arytenoid cartilage resection as needed. Additionally, cancer excision at the anterior commissure must include excision of the perichondrium, and in some cases resection of the thyroid cartilage itself. Additionally, the inferior extent of cancer extension must be meticulously determined endoscopically to preclude cancer escape in the area of the cricothyroid membrane. CO_2 laser resection of stage II glottic cancer in appropriately selected patients is an important addition to the surgical techniques available to the head and neck oncologist.

References

1   Vaughan CW, Strong MS, Jako GJ: Laryngeal carcinoma: Transoral treatment utilizing the CO_2 laser. Am J Surg 1978;136:490–493.
2   Davis RK, Jako GJ, Hyams VJ, Shapshay SM: The anatomical limitations of CO_2 laser cordectomy. Laryngoscope 1982;92:980–984.
3   Blakeslee D, Vaughan CW, Shapshay SM, et al: Excisional biopsy in the selected management of T1 glottic cancer: A three-year follow-up study. Laryngoscope 1984;94:488–494.
4   Davis RK, Kelly SM, Parkin JL, Stevens MH, Johnson LP: Selective management of early glottic cancer. Laryngoscope 1990;100:1306–1309.
5   McGuirt WF, Koufman JA: Endoscopic laser surgery. Arch Otolaryngol Head Neck Surg 1987;113:501–505.
6   Wetmore SJ, Key M, Suen JY: Laser therapy for T1 glottic carcinoma of the larynx. Arch Otolaryngol Head Neck Surg 1986;112:853–855.
7   Kelly MD, Hahn SS, Spaulding CA, Kersh CR, Constable WC, Cantrell RW: Definitive radiotherapy in the management of stage I and II carcinomas of the glottis. Ann Otolrhinollaryngol 1989;98:235–239.
8   Howell-Burke D, Peters LJ, Goepfert H, Oswald MJ: T2 glottic cancer. Recurrence, salvage and survival after definitive radiotherapy. Arch Otolaryngol Head Neck Surg 1990;116:830–835.
9   Pellitteri PK, Kennedy TL, Vrabec DP, Beiler D, Hellstrom M: Radiotherapy in the mainstay in the treatment of early glottic carcinoma. Arch Otolaryngol Head Neck Surg 1991;117:297–301.
10 Ton-Van J, Lefebure JL, Stern JC, Buisset E, Coche-Dequeant B, VanKemmel B: Comparison of surgery and radiotherapy in T1 and T2 glottic carcinomas. Am J Surg 1991;162:337–340.
11 Steiner W: Results of curative laser microsurgery of laryngeal carcinoma. Am J Otolaryngol 1993;14:116–121.

R. Kim Davis, MD, Division of Otolaryngology, Head and Neck Surgery,
John A. Dixon Laser Institute, University of Utah School of Medicine,
50 N. Medical Drive, Room 3C120, Salt Lake City, UT 84132 (USA)

Subject Index

wavelength effect on injury 23, 24
light absorption 23
protection of operating staff 24, 25

Fibronectin, lack in laser wounds 13
Fluorescence, measurement in tumors
49–52

Gingival hyperplasia, removal by lasers
137, 138
Ginkgo extract, treatment with soft-laser
for tinnitus
efficacy 102–104, 106–108
extract dose 105, 106
laser
light administration 106
transmission measurement 107
long-term effects 103
mechanism of laser action 105
Glottic cancer
arytenoid cartilage invasion 257
radiotherapy 255, 256
transoral laser excision
biopsy 255
endoscopy 256, 257
limitations 254
local control rate 257
outcome 255

Hemangioma, *see also* Port wine stain
classification 67, 70, 71
differential diagnosis 72, 73
incidence at birth 70, 71
involution rate 72
MRI 68
natural history 71, 72, 79
treatment
goals 68
laser treatment
carbon dioxide laser 133
cooling techniques 75, 76, 79
Nd:YAG laser 68, 69, 73, 75–79, 85
yellow light laser 73–75
scarring 68, 69
steroid therapy 73
Hematoporphyrin derivative
components 44, 48

efficacy 59
excitation band 44, 53
photodynamic therapy 31, 32, 36, 40, 44,
53, 58–60
skin phototoxicity 34, 36, 39, 44, 48, 59
tissue selectivity 46, 48, 59
Hemoglobin, absorption of laser light 5
Ho:YAG laser
delivery systems 122
turbinate reduction surgery 122, 123
Hypopharyngeal diverticulum, *see*
Zenker's diverticulum

Interferon, papilloma therapy
duration of treatment 166
effectiveness with laser surgery 166–168
side effects 162,166

Keratinocyte, laser wound effect on
migration 13

Laryngeal cancer, *see also* Anterior
commissure, Glottic cancer, Supraglottic
carcinoma, Vocal cords
imaging
anterior commissure 208
arytenoid cartilage invasion 209
cricothyreoid membrane 210
CT 207–211
MRI 207–211
reliability 210, 211
supraglottic cancer 209
thyroid cartilage invasion 209
laser surgery 155
classification 212–214
indications 213, 245
transoral resection, recurrence rate
246, 248, 251, 252
metastasis 248
radiotherapy 250–252
tumor staging 212, 213
Laser, *see* Argon laser, Carbon dioxide
laser, Er:YAG laser, Ho:YAG laser,
Nd:YAG laser
Laser plume
content
bacteria 16, 18

Port wine stain
  laser treatment 82, 83
  natural history 72, 73

Radiation therapy
  glottic cancer 255, 256
  laryngeal cancer 250–252
  supraglottic cancer 230, 232, 234, 235,
    238, 239
  vocal cord preservation 215, 219, 226
Ranula, excision by lasers 133, 137

Salivary duct stones, lithotripsy with dye
    laser
  endoscope 149, 151
  fragmentation rate 148
  laser operation 149, 150
  lithotripter 149
  outcome 150–152
  patient selection 149
Stapedotomy
  acoustic impulse from lasers 89–92, 97,
    98
  heat generation by lasers 89–91, 96, 97
  operating parameters of carbon dioxide
    lasers 99, 100
  perforation of stapes base by lasers 87–89
Supraglottic carcinoma
  imaging 209
  laser surgery
    endoscopy
      indications 231
      morbidity 233
      neck dissection 232, 234, 235
      outcome 233–235
      radiotherapy 232, 234, 235
      resection 232
    partial resection
      advantages over endolaryngeal
        technique 243
      indications 241
      laryngofissure access 241, 242
      outcome 242, 243
      postoperative care 244
      postoperative functional recovery
        237–239
      radiotherapy 238, 239

transoral
  contraindications 228
  laryngoscope 227, 228
  laser settings 227
  outcome 229, 230
  postoperative recovery 237–239
  radiotherapy 230
  tumor excision 228

Tattoo removal, argon laser technique 63
Telangiectasias, laser treatment 84
Thermal damage
  carbonization 1, 9
  effect on histological examination of
    leukoplakia 128
  necrosis 11
  prevention 68, 75, 76
  temperature effect on tissue 1
Tinnitus, treatment with soft-laser/Ginkgo
    extract
  efficacy 102–104, 106–108
  extract dose 105, 106
  laser
    light administration 106
    transmission measurement 107
  long-term effects 103
  mechanism of laser action 105
Tonsils, hyperplastic lingual
  associated diseases 156
  laser surgery
    complications 154, 156
    indications 130, 131
    lymphoma 153, 154
    postoperative care 154
    success rate 130, 131, 154–156
Tracheal stenosis, granulation removal by
    lase surgery
  ArthroLase™ guide system 180, 181
  indications 179
  outcome 180, 181
Turbinate
  reduction surgery
    carbon dioxide laser
      complications 120
      laser settings 118, 120
      postoperative evaluation 119
    Ho:YAG laser 122, 123

Turbinate (cont.)
    treatment for hyperplasia 118–120
Tympanostomy, acoustic impulse from
    lasers 92

Ultrasonography, tumor examination 49

Venous lakes, laser treatment 84
Vocal cords
    bilateral nerve paralysis
        conventional surgery 170, 174, 176
        etiology 170, 171, 182
        laser artaenoidectomy
            effect on air flow 173, 183
            endoscopic suturing 172
            Kashima's technique 174, 175
            Kleinsasser technique 177, 178,
                183, 245
            outcome 171–173, 175, 177, 178,
                182, 183
            postoperative care 183
            tracheostomy 176
        posterior chordectomy 177, 178
    laser resection of carcinomas
        carbon dioxide laser settings 219, 222,
            224
        healing time 219, 221
        indications 219
        metastasis 224, 226

outcome 220
recurrence rate 224, 226
tumor excision 222, 224
laser surgery for benign lesions
    anesthesia 158
    indications 158, 159
    outcomes 159
radiation therapy for preservation 215,
    219, 226
vascularization of lesions 158
voice preservation in surgery
    evaluation 215–218
    laser artaenoidectomy 171–173, 175
    laser cordectomy 216–218
    partial resection 216, 218

Wound healing
    laser-induced delay 9, 11, 13, 65, 157
    phases
        exudative 8, 9
        proliferate 8, 9
        repair 8, 9

Zenker's diverticulum, laser microendos-
    copy 140–143
    coagulation 140, 142
    complications 141, 142
    postoperative care 140, 141

Trends in Language Acquisition Research

Official publication of the International Association
for the Study of Child Language (IASCL).
IASCL website: http://atila-www.uia.ac.be/IASCL

Series Editors

Annick De Houwer
University of Antwerp/UIA
annick.dehouwer@ua.ac.be

Steven Gillis
University of Antwerp/UIA
steven.gillis@ua.ac.be

Advisory Board

Jean Berko Gleason
Boston University

Ruth Berman
Tel Aviv University

Philip Dale
University of Missouri-Columbia

Paul Fletcher
Hong Kong University

Brian MacWhinney
Carnegie Mellon University

Volume 2
Directions in Sign Language Acquisition
Edited by Gary Morgan and Bencie Woll

Directions in Sign Language Acquisition